Rehabilitation
Institute of
Chicago
PROCEDURE
MANUAL

SPINAL CORD INJURY

A GUIDE TO FUNCTIONAL OUTCOMES IN PHYSICAL THERAPY MANAGEMENT

Vickie Nixon, P.T.

Frederick Schneider, M.Ed., P.T.
Physical Therapy Series Editor

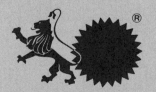

AN ASPEN PUBLICATION®

Aspen Publishers, Inc.
Rockville, Maryland
1985

Library of Congress Cataloging in Publication Data

Nixon, Vickie.
Spinal cord injury.

"An Aspen publication."
Bibliography: p. 225.
Includes index.
1. Spinal cord—Wounds and injuries—Patients—Rehabilitation. 2. Physical therapy.
I. Rehabilitation Institute of Chicago.
II. Title. [DNLM: 1. Physical Therapy—methods—handbooks.
2. Spinal Cord Injuries—rehabilitation—handbooks. WL39N736s]
RD594.3.N59 1985 617'.482044 84-18474
ISBN: 0-89443-552-3

Editorial Services: M. Eileen Higgins

Library of Congress Catalog Card Number: 84-18474
ISBN: 0-89443-552-3

Printed in the United States of America

8 9

Table of Contents

Series Preface

The three guides that comprise this series are outgrowths of procedural manuals used in the physical therapy department at the Rehabilitation Institute of Chicago. These manuals originated when the Institute was established in 1954, and when the department initially consisted of only one therapist: Hildegarde Myers. The first few pages of protocols that addressed the Institute's three most common diagnostic groups (stroke/head injury, amputation, and spinal cord injury) multiplied as the department grew. A few years ago, a committee was formed to reorganize this now large volume of material into concise and uniform formats by using tables to outline the rehabilitation outcomes expected for patients with one of these three clinical problems.

It was subsequently decided to rewrite the three manuals into a format suitable for distribution and use outside the Institute. We reached this decision based on our observation of the use of these manuals by interns and new staff. These individuals, in most instances, had come to the Institute with strong theoretical backgrounds and baseline competencies in clinical skills. What they lacked was the ability to enter into the "process" of clinical problem-solving. Our contention is that clinical interns and new graduates need a framework from which to develop this "process of problem-solving." To us at the Institute, this "process" is the mark of a well qualified physical therapy practitioner. By incorporating this "process" into charts, we hope to assist clinicians in referencing during treatment planning. Each guide is designed to answer the question: "Have I considered all aspects in managing this patient?" Finally, we feel that the students and clinicians who use these guides during affiliations and the initial periods of practice will be far ahead of others; their path to more advanced clinical learning (such as the ability to analyze and compare aspects of evaluation and treatment) will be accelerated.

It is the intent of the Institute that these three texts present: (1.) the "process" for determining comprehensive physical therapy management of patients with one of the three clinical problems; (2.) a systematic clinical problem-solving approach to treatment planning; and (3.) equipment and treatment ideas based on experience and observations of a large number of clinicians. These texts focus on what functional outcomes can be expected with various degrees of disability found with each of the three clinical situations. Management is then analyzed in terms of these functional outcomes.

As the reader regards the Institute's stated opinions on the efficacy of specific equipment, he or she should note that these opinions are based on the experiences of the Institute's department staff and not on statistical data. These opinions do not constitute an endorsement of equipment. Discussions of the pros and cons of equipment are provided as a tool for therapists so that they might more effectively manage their patients.

FREDERICK J. SCHNEIDER, M.ED., P.T.

Director, Physical Therapy Education
Physical Therapy Series Editor
Rehabilitation Institute of Chicago
Chicago, Illinois

Preface

This guide is written primarily for the therapist who is new to the treatment of the SCI patient. The information presented is not necessarily new, but is perhaps organized differently from other texts. The first part of the guide deals with the SCI patient in a general way, discussing the evaluation process, setting general goals, and creating general treatment programs. In the second part, some specific outcomes are discussed in more detail. Each unit in this section includes outcome charts for specific levels of injury, equipment recommendations, and a general discussion of the various treatment approaches for that goal.

Because it is assumed that the therapist does not just follow a ''cookbook'' approach to exercises, a fairly traditional problem-solving outline has been followed. The cycle of evaluation⟶goal setting⟶treatment planning⟶treatment⟶evaluation . . . is emphasized.

This guide has been designed as a treatment resource. The Institute's therapists believe that a therapist's best learning occurs when he or she deals with real life problems. Therefore, the reader may wish to skip the information on ambulation until he or she is actually working with an ambulatory patient. The guide's information on the quadriplegic patient will seem practical only to those who are working with quadriplegic patients; otherwise, the information could seem academic. The guide should be used as a resource to help a beginning therapist solve specific problems encountered in patient treatment.

Finally, the Institute's therapists believe that the most effective treatment with SCI patients is found in the team approach. The physical therapist is only one member of this team. Some references to the other team members are made throughout the guide. However, it is often assumed that the physical therapist will seek out the assistance of other team members as needed to maximize their goals in patient treatment.

Vicki Nixon, P.T.

Supervisor, Physical Therapy Department
Rehabilitation Institute of Chicago
Chicago, Illinois

Acknowledgments

One clinician in our physical therapy department assumed responsibility for compiling and writing each of the three guides. The content of these guides, however, is based on the experiences and contributions of the many therapists who have worked in our clinical department. Most notable among them are: *Ann Charness, Mary Massery, Jane Sullivan,* and *Toni Tait-Baer* in the spinal cord injury guide; *Bonnie Buol, May Cotterman, Ellen Ferris, Deborah Jevey-Young, Patricia Kammerer,* and *Melanie Moody* in the amputee guide; and *Ellen Gilbert* and *Deborah Shefrin* in the stroke/head trauma guide.

The Institute would like to thank *Ruth Ann Watkins,* Vice President for Allied Health Services at the Institute, for her review of the manuscripts and ensuing helpful suggestions. Also deserving of thanks are *Henry B. Betts, M.D.,* Medical Director and Vice Chairman of the Institute, and *Don A. Olson, Ph.D.,* Director of Academic Development at the Institute, for their valuable assistance in gaining the initial funding for this project.

Special appreciation is extended to *Oscar Izquierdo,* who took the photographs for all three guides, and to the patients and students who gave of their time to pose for these pictures. We also thank *Catherine Finnegan* and *Linda Ruben* for typing and proofreading the manuscripts; and *Mary Tanabe Moy* and *Leatrice Campbell* for their assistance in word processing.

Finally, this project gained its initial impetus through funding provided in part by the Esmark, Inc. Foundation.

Aids to Using the Guide

ABBREVIATIONS

The following abbreviations have been used:

ADL	Activities of daily living
AFO	Ankle-foot orthosis
BFO	Balanced forearm orthosis
COG	Center of gravity
FES	Functional electrical stimulation
GPB	Glossopharyngeal breathing
KAFO	Knee-ankle-foot orthosis
MMT	Manual muscle test
OT	Occupational therapist
PT	Physical therapist
ROM	Range of motion
SCI	Spinal cord injury, spinal cord injured
SOMI	Sterno-occipital mandibular immobilization
TLSO	Thoracic-lumbar-sacral orthosis
VC	Vital capacity
W/C	Wheelchair

DEFINITION OF TERMS

Ankle-foot orthosis (AFO)—an orthopedic appliance or apparatus; in this case, a short leg brace

Anterior cord syndrome—incomplete lesion. Damage is mainly in the anterior cord so the senses of light touch, proprioception, and position are usually preserved.

Autonomic hyperreflexia—exaggerated autonomic responses to stimuli (e.g., stimulus: distended bladder; response: pounding headache, profuse sweating above level of lesion, severe hypertension, bradycardia)

Brown-Séquard syndrome—incomplete lesion. Complete loss of motor function on same side as lesion with loss of pain and temperature senses on the opposite side. Functionally, the limb with the best motor control has the poorest sensation.

Central cord syndrome—incomplete lesion in which greater deficits are found in the more centrally located cervical tracts (arms) than peripherally located lumbar and sacral tracts (legs)

Compensatory movement patterns—patterns of movement used to accommodate for absent or weak musculature

Compensatory sensory techniques—techniques used to compensate for sensory deficits

Complete lesion—no sensation or voluntary muscle power below the neurological level of the lesion

Controlled mobility—ability to move proximal segment over fixed distal segments

Equilibrium reactions—automatic reactions that serve to maintain or restore balance during activity, especially when in danger of falling; ability to regain one's COG

Expiratory reserve volume—the extra volume of air exhaled during prolonged or forced expiration

Functional component skills—elementary skills needed to perform complex functional activity (i.e., head control is a functional component skill needed for sitting balance)

Glossopharyngeal breathing (GPB)—a technique used to increase VC. Air is essentially "sucked" into the lungs.

Halo—one method of external stabilization of cervical vertebrae

Harrington rods—method used to provide internal stabilization for thoracic and lumbar vertebrae

Heterotopic ossification (ectopic or hypertrophic bone)—abnormal laying down of bone across joints. The hip, knee, elbow, and shoulder joints are most frequently involved.

Incomplete lesion—sensation or voluntary muscle power below the neurological level of the lesion

Inspiratory reserve volume—the extra volume of air needed for prolonged or forced inspiration

Jewett orthosis (TLSO)—method of providing external stabilization to thoracic and lumbar vertebrae

Kinesthetic awareness—awareness of body position and movement in space

Knee-ankle-foot orthosis (KAFO)—an orthopedic appliance or apparatus; in this case, a long leg brace

Knight-Taylor orthosis (TLSO)—method of providing external stabilization to thoracic and lumbar vertebrae

Lesion level—the most distal uninvolved cord segment (e.g., C7 complete would mean that the patient had impaired or absent sensation and/or voluntary muscle power below the C7 segment)

Long sitting—sitting with knees extended

Mild increase in tone—some resistance to passive stretch is noted, but increases in tone do not interfere with ROM or function.

Moderate increase in tone—more resistance to passive stretch is noted, and increase in tone may make ranging more difficult; however, ROM remains within normal limits. Patient will still be able to perform the ADL, but the quality of the performance may be impaired.

Momentum—the product of a body's mass and linear velocity

Motor skills—that which is necessary to impart motion (i.e., ROM, strength, sensation)

Outcome—goal; performance expectation

Process—steps necessary to achieve the outcome

Protective extension reaction—ability to prevent the head from hitting the ground after COG has been displaced to the point where it can no longer be regained

Quad systems wheelchair—electric W/C that is both electrically propelled and reclined

Sacral sparing—incomplete lesion in which sensation is intact in the sacral area. Paralysis and loss of sensation are complete in all other areas below lesion level.

Severe increase in tone—tone is increased to the point where ROM can no longer be maintained within normal limits. ADL will be decreased secondary to tone.

Short sitting—sitting with knees flexed over the edge of a mat, bed, etc.

Significant other—close friends and/or family members of the SCI patient

Skill—ability to fix proximal segment and move distal parts

Stability—ability to maintain a posture

Sterno-occipital mandibular immobilization (SOMI)—one method of external stabilizing of cervical vertebrae

Thoracic-lumbar-sacral orthosis (TLSO)—any orthosis that provides external immobilization of the thoracic and lumbar spine

Tidal volume—air displaced between normal inspiration and expiration

UCB/NYU orthotic shoe insert—shoe insert with ankle joint developed by the University of California at Berkeley and New York University

Vital capacity (VC)—tidal volume plus inspiratory and expiratory reserve volumes

Weiss springs—method of providing internal stabilization for thoracic and lumbar vertebrae

EXPLANATION OF OUTCOME CHARTS

This guide includes many charts (divided into three columns) outlining specific expectations for the SCI patient. These charts are only meant to act as guides. A patient's progress should never be limited by a therapist whose expectations are too low. While the therapist's expectations need to be realistic, he or she also needs to understand that often the patients will do more if more is expected: many patients fail to meet their maximum potential simply because the therapist expects too little. Each patient should always be challenged to meet the maximum potential.

The purpose of the *Outcome* column is to describe the expected level of safe function for the SCI patient. The outcomes suggested in this text are based on the clinical observations of physical therapists at the Rehabilitation Institute of Chicago. As needed, outcomes are further defined under the subheading *Components*.

Not all patients will be able to achieve the stated outcomes. Some will even surpass the levels of function suggested. This is why the *Considerations* column is included. Listed here are factors that may interfere with or, in some cases, aid in the accomplishment of the outcome. The list is not inclusive. Only those considerations that are particularly relevant to the outcome are stated. For instance, associated medical problems and psychological status are rarely listed, even though, when present, these certainly have a bearing on most outcomes.

The third column outlines the *Process* used to achieve the outcome. Again, the intent is not to include

every possible step in the process but rather to suggest a systematic approach to treatment planning.

An outcome summary is presented in Appendix A.

Please note that these charts are meant to be working guides for use when working with specific patients and not necessarily something to be read word for word in one sitting. This is why many of the items in each column of the specific outcomes are repeated from one injury level to the next. In an effort to make these more useful, any changes made from the previous level have been put in italics. For instance, if *tone* is listed as a consideration for the C6 quadriplegic, but was not listed for the C5 quadriplegic, it will be put in italics the first time it is listed in the consideration column for the C6 quadriplegic.

EQUIPMENT INTRODUCTION AND EXPLANATION OF CHARTS

Included in any definition of independence for the SCI patient is equipment that may be needed. Because of this, much of the data on ADL includes some discussion of equipment options. The information presented in the charts illustrates a process that might be useful in deciding which equipment to use. Some of the issues that need consideration are outlined in one column, and comments and observations made by former patients and staff at the Rehabilitation Institute of Chicago regarding the various products listed are presented in other columns. These comments should be viewed only as examples of things to consider. The intent is not to recommend a particular piece of equipment but rather to use familiar equipment to illustrate a process of decision making.

Neither the list of issues to be considered nor the comments made on individual companies and their products is meant to be exhaustive. The information in the charts is only meant to be a starting point. Cost and delivery time are just two examples of other issues that should be considered and yet are not covered in this guide because of their variability.

It should also be understood that while many of the issues listed will always need consideration, many of the specific comments made regarding these issues will become obsolete with time. It is the responsibility of each individual involved in equipment decisions to accurately reflect the current market to their patients. Equipment companies, especially those making W/Cs, are more competitive than they ever have been in the past. The market is changing daily; what's true today may not be true tomorrow.

Equipment available in one area is not always as available in other areas. In addition, each area has different environmental demands, necessitating different life styles that create different equipment needs. Because of this, no attempt has been made to discuss every piece of equipment on the market. Many other comparable products already exist and many more will exist in the future.

The equipment discussed in this guide is that which is most available to the Rehabilitation Institute of Chicago, is readily obtained, and is easily maintained. It is that which we have found to provide the most accessibility, mobility, durability, and safety with our patient population. No endorsement or exclusion of products is intended.

Guidelines to Equipment Prescription

Like all other decisions the best solutions will only be found if an organized approach is taken. The following is an example of a process that might be used.

Involve the Patient

Even though the therapist has a professional responsibility to third party payers to accurately reflect the medical needs of the patient regarding equipment recommendations, the therapist should place much of the onus for equipment decisions on the patient. After all, it is the patient who will have to use the equipment for the next five to ten years.

Granted, this does not always seem to be the quickest and easiest way to approach this problem. Few people are able to make their best decisions in the midst of such a devastating crisis. In addition, many have experienced the world outside of the rehabilitation facility as a disabled individual only on weekends, at best. Ideally, in order to make the best decision, a patient needs time to adjust to the disability and learn what it is like to live in the world as a disabled person. Too frequently, however, our systems do not allow for this luxury of time.

This leads many well-intentioned therapists to make equipment decisions *for* their patients. By doing this they rob the patient of a valuable opportunity to learn problem solving skills; additionally, the therapists are just not able to make the best decision alone.

The best decisions can only be made if the therapist and patient work together. The therapist's job is to provide the patient with the tools needed to solve problems. The therapist's past experience with other patients and pieces of equipment can be a valuable resource file for the patient. The therapist can introduce the patient to other disabled peers and offer exposure to various approaches to ADL that will be essential to the patient's decision-making process. If this is done, the patient will then be more prepared to make the final decisions on the equipment.

Outline All ADL That Will Impact on the Equipment Items Being Considered

In considering a W/C, for instance, one needs to consider not only how well it performs in getting from point A to point B, but also how easily pressure relief maneuvers can be managed and how transfers and often assumption of standing can be accomplished.

Establish Other Factors That Will Be Important To the Patient

Such factors as cost, durability, comfort, accessibility, and so on should be considered.

Establish Patient Priorities

What ADL skills are critical? What other equipment qualities are most important (e.g., cost, durability, comfort)? No piece of equipment will ever be able to give a patient everything desired. In addition, funding is usually not unlimited. Compromises will always have to be made.

Explore the Market

The charts provided in the ADL chapters are one example of how to approach this task.

Set Up a Trial Period with the Possible Equipment Options

Make Final Decisions

Decide on equipment and resolve specific prescription fit issues (e.g., how wide should the W/C be?).

Finally, since equipment is discussed throughout this guide, the following considerations should be kept in mind:

Before making equipment decisions . . .

- perform a thorough evaluation of motor skills, estimate potential daily living status/functional skills, do a home assessment, and finalize discharge plans. Include information from all team members.

- always consider equipment for the individual patient. Needs and abilities vary with the level of function (not necessarily the level of lesion), the environment (home, school, work, nursing home), and the patient's life style. Patient consent is necessary; however, it is important to prescribe what the patient needs, not necessarily the equipment that the patient wants. Maintain professional integrity by not abusing funds or prescribing equipment that will not be used.

- be familiar with reliable equipment vendors in the area who will allow trial periods on equipment in the department and introduce new equipment, who provide prompt and accurate deliveries of orders, and who provide good maintenance and repair of equipment provided.

- be familiar with the rules and regulations of third party payers and alternative funding resources available from private interest groups or free funding services of hospitals. For example, some Medicare and Medicaid regulations prohibit funding for electrical equipment (beds and W/Cs) or consider some equipment to be luxury items. Some health interest societies and foundations have stores of equipment that they will lend to the patient for limited or indefinite periods.

Do not . . .

- prescribe equipment if it, or at least a reasonable facsimile, has not been tried. Do not guess at sizes or estimate safety. Ask questions about dimensions, layouts, and styles of fixtures in the home. Preferably, give a home assessment form (Appendix F, Exhibit F–4) to the patient to complete before any equipment is ordered.

- prescribe expensive definitive equipment if the patient's status is changing or if he is being sent to a rehabilitation facility. Rental equipment is a good alternative for a limited time and will save money and problems in the long run. Replacing accessories or entire pieces of equipment is very costly, and, if extra funding is not approved, the patient may have trouble functioning with inadequate equipment.

Evaluation

One of the first steps in any planning process is data collection. Information needs to be gathered from the patient and his physical examination, as well as from his medical charts, his family and friends, and other team members. This step provides the therapist with the information needed to develop realistic and meaningful outcomes.

Data collection is not, however, the only function of an evaluation. It should also function as a teaching tool. The patient needs to learn what is being evaluated and why. Without this information, problem solving later on in his rehabilitation stay will be more difficult. This is one of the patient's first opportunities to become actively involved in his rehabilitation process and unless he is involved at this point, it will be much more difficult to get him involved later. Treatment does not start after the evaluation is completed. Evaluation is a very integral part of the entire treatment process.

New and different evaluation procedures, specifically for the SCI patient, do not exist. One must still look at strength, ROM, and sensation, and these procedures should be familiar. In addition, all therapists understand the need to maintain objectivity and limit the subjectivity inevitably present whenever an evaluation is done, and all realize that the validity of their observations will depend on their consistency as evaluators, their method of evaluation, and the instruments used. However, the implications of the patient deficits found during an evaluation may not be as well understood. The following outline highlights some of these implications:

I. PHYSICAL EVALUATION

A. Skin

1. Process to include:
   a. Special note of more vulnerable skin over bony prominences
   b. Scar tissue that breaks down more easily
2. Implications to patient care:
   a. Pressure sores may limit the postures and positions available during treatment.
   b. Training and treatment are often delayed.
   c. A patient may become frustrated with training delays and bored with limited treatment techniques. Motivation therefore may be decreased.
   d. Because of the high risk in this patient population for potential skin problems, preventive measures become very important.

B. Sensory

1. Process to include:
   a. All sensory areas (e.g., pain and temperature, light touch, proprioception)

b. Evaluation of a patient's awareness of his deficits

c. Evaluation of a patient's ability to compensate for his deficits

2. Implications for patient care:

a. Bruises, burns, and so on are more likely to occur with decreased sensory feedback.

b. Deficits may impair coordination, making self-care and ADL more difficult.

c. Learning new motor skills may take longer because of decreased feedback.

d. A patient's sensory warning systems are no longer intact. At least initially, therefore, he no longer has the freedom to be as spontaneous and impetuous as he may have been prior to injury.

e. Skin condition must be closely monitored with the use of any adaptive equipment, such as splinting, bracing, and other aids.

f. Frequent pressure relief maneuvers will need to be added to the patient's daily routine to accommodate decreased ischial and sacral sensation.

g. More careful attention will have to be focused on items (if any) that are placed in back pants pockets and to clothing in general. Things like thick seams and tight shoes can contribute to pressure sore development.

C. Respiration (see Appendix F, Exhibit F-3)

1. General observations

a. Process to include:

(1) Notation of:

(a) Patient's color

(b) Chest formation, shape, symmetry, bony abnormalities, and so on

(c) Muscle tone

(d) Muscle atrophy

(e) Presence of artificial airways (tracheostomy or any type of tube)

(2) Review of significant respiratory treatment and other associated medical problems

b. Implications for patient care:

(1) Chest formation, shape, and symmetry can indicate possible muscle weakness and decreased chest mobility.

(2) Respiratory history and associated medical problems may indicate the need for more intensive preventive education.

2. ROM

a. Process to include:

(1) Evaluation of upper and lower chest expansion and mobility, measured below nipple line and at xiphoid processes. Note any asymmetries present.

(2) Evaluation of changes in chest expansion with air shifts and GPB

(3) Evaluation of motions available at other body joints, particularly at shoulders, hips, and trunk

b. Implications for patient care:

(1) Decreased chest expansion and mobility can decrease VC. Normally chest expansion is two and one-half to three inches at xiphoid process.

(2) Normal ROM at shoulders will facilitate greater chest expansion. If the patient has enough shoulder extension to position the upper extremities behind the push handle of a W/C, for instance, he will fix the pectoral girdle, facilitating greater action of accessory muscles on the chest wall, and increase chest expansion, especially of the upper anterior portion.

(3) Flexion of trunk and hips in sitting position can be used in assistive coughing techniques. Without normal ROM, these techniques cannot be used.

(4) Back posture, which includes the normal cervical, thoracic, and lumbar curves, facilitates respiration. Excessive tightness in the trunk extensors or abdominal muscles will preclude this good posture. The optimal positioning of ribs, which allows for maximal chest expansion, occurs when these normal curves are present.

3. Respiratory muscle strength (Figure 1–1)

a. Process to include:

(1) Evaluation of diaphragm (C3–C5)

(2) Evaluation of abdominal muscles (T5–T12)

(3) Evaluation of accessory muscles

(a) Intercostals (T1–T12). Elevates the ribs, creating lateral costal expansion, and maintains the integrity of the intercostal spaces.

(b) Pectorals (C5–T1) are used with forced inspiration when the arms are fixed. The contraction of this muscle causes upper chest, primarily anterior, expansion.

  (c) Serratus (C5–C7). If scapula is fixed, these muscle fibers act to increase posterior expansion.

  (d) Scalenes (C3–C8). Contraction increases upper chest, primarily superior expansion.

  (e) Sternocleidomastoid and upper trapezius (cranial nerve IX and C1–C4). If head is fixed, the sternum is elevated as the muscles contract.

  (f) Erector spinae (C1 and down). Extends vertebral column in deep inspiration, allowing for further sternal elevation.

b. Implications for patient care:

  (1) Absence of abdominal muscles may severely impair a cough owing to inability to build up intrathoracic pressure to expel the air forcefully; bronchial hygiene may then be inadequate.

  (2) Adaptive equipment may be indicated to facilitate increased VC:

    (a) An abdominal binder may be used to substitute for the abdominal muscles.

    (b) Trunk supports on W/C may provide the added trunk stability needed for chest mobility.

  (3) Posture will play a much greater role in respiration. Normally breathing is done most efficiently when sitting because the abdominal contents are pushed up against the diaphragm and allow for greater excursion of movement. The SCI patient breathes best when lying supine because the abdominal contents lie closer to the diaphragm and push it up; therefore, the diaphragm has a fulcrum to act against. Gravity and the weight of the abdominal contents replace paralyzed abdominal muscles and help to position the diaphragm for maximal lateral costal and inferior expansion. When the patient begins to sit up, the abdominal contents will fall. Diaphragm exertion is decreased, being limited to inferior excursion only. Therefore, the

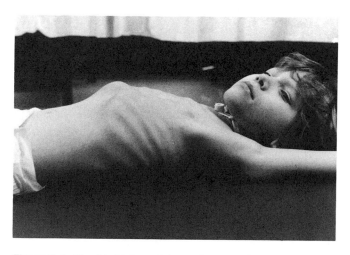

Figure 1–1 Atrophied intercostal muscles are pulled into the chest cavity during inspiration.

change in intrathoracic pressure is decreased and the patient takes in less air. This is why many new patients complain of shortness of breath when sitting. The supine position has other advantages for the SCI patient. Since the effects of gravity are eliminated and the spine is stabilized against the bed, even weak accessory muscles will be able to assist with breathing in this position.

4. Quiet respiration

a. Process to include:

  (1) Analysis of muscles and breathing patterns (should be made in several different positions)

  (2) Evaluation of tidal volume (should be approximately four cubic centimeters per pound of body weight, or one tenth of VC)

  (3) Evaluation of respiratory rate (in breaths per minute; usually remains unchanged even without a normal diaphragm, being 12 to 20 breaths per minute)

  (4) Evaluation of phonation skills (usually eight to ten syllables per breath)

  (5) Evaluation of coordination of breathing with functional activities

  (6) Evaluation of augmented breathing skills, such as GPB

b. Implications for patient care:

  (1) If diaphragm is weak, use of accessory muscles may be seen.

  (2) Tidal volume for the normal adult is 450 to 600 ml. At least 150 ml of air is

needed for the air to reach the alveoli. A decrease in tidal volume means that a greater percentage of each breath is ventilating "dead" space (e.g., nose, mouth, pharynx, trachea) and less is getting to the alveoli. The work of breathing is increased, and less energy is left for other functional activities.

(3) Increased respiratory rate may indicate shallow breaths. Ventilation to lower lobes is decreased, increasing the likelihood of infection.

(4) If patient is *hypoventilating,* he may exhibit drowsiness and irritability. Appetite may decrease; arousal from sleep may be difficult in the morning, perhaps because oxygen levels are lower. (Note: This frequently happens with the quadriplegic with a high-level injury because he cannot use his accessory muscles while sleeping, since this is a conscious act.)

(5) With *hyperventilation,* the patient may experience faintness, tingling, and numbness.

(6) Decreased phonation skills may impair a patient's ability to direct his care (decreased eccentric control of the diaphragm).

(7) Poor coordination of breathing with functional activities will decrease endurance.

(8) GPB increases inspiratory capability, which will improve a cough and overall ventilation of the various lobes, decreasing the possibility of respiratory complications.

5. Bronchial hygiene
   a. Process to include:
      (1) Evaluation of cough (force, timing, sound, productivity)
      (2) Evaluation of VC (for predicted standard values see Morris, J.F. et al. in bibliography); VC, both with and without augmented breathing patterns, should be considered.
      (3) Evaluation of patient's knowledge of and ability to assume (and/or direct) postural drainage positions.
      (4) Evaluation of patient's comfort level with movement

b. Implications for patient care:
   (1) VC may be used as a baseline to define weakness of respiratory muscles.
   (2) Decreased VC may mean decreased cough effectiveness and necessitate teaching of assistive cough techniques to patient and/or family.
   (3) Postural drainage and the ability to cough take on greater significance with the SCI patient. These patients are often dependent, which increases the possibility of secretion pooling and thus infection.
   (4) The more comfortable the patient is with movement, the more likely it is that he will move or ask someone to move him. Movement decreases the possibility of secretion pooling and thus infection.

D. ROM

1. Process to include:
   a. Complete evaluation of all motions available at each joint
   b. Considerations for selective tightness in some muscles:
      (1) Low back
      (2) Hamstrings (no more than 110 degrees needed)
      (3) Long finger flexors
2. Difficulties to anticipate in testing:
   a. Immobilization devices (e.g., SOMI, Halo, TLSO) often limit full ROM. Positioning may be difficult. Accuracy may then be decreased.
   b. Pain
3. Implications for patient care:
   a. ADL. Because extremes in range often play important roles in compensating for strength deficits, decreases in ROM at almost any joint can make major differences in the level of independence. Listed below are some key joint ranges and their functional significance:
      (1) Shoulder flexion, abduction, and external rotation
         (a) Frequently limited in quadriplegic patients because of immobilization devices.
         (b) Important for transfers (e.g., prone-on-elbows push and swivel bar

transfers—see Chapter 8) and upper extremity dressing

    (2) Shoulder extension

        (a) Frequently limited because of difficulties in ranging during acute phases

        (b) Particularly important motion for the quadriplegic who uses it to assist in providing a stable sitting position in the W/C (hooking arms behind W/C push handles)

        (c) Needed for the supine-on-elbows posture, which is a preliminary posture to many higher level skills

        (d) Can be combined with external rotation to give the quadriplegic patient the ability to lock his elbows and maintain long sitting with upper extremity support

    (3) Hip and knee flexion and rotation

        (a) Needed for lower extremity dressing

        (b) Needed for transfers (goal should be at least 90 degrees of hip flexion; however, a quadriplegic will probably need more than 90 degrees of hip flexion)

    (4) Hip and knee extension—for functional ambulation

    (5) Ankle dorsiflexion (at least to neutral)

b. Selective tightness of the low back musculature and hamstrings provides the quadriplegic with an easier method of maintaining long sitting balance. With tightness he is essentially able to hang on the muscles and balance without using extra muscle power.

c. In addition to making long sitting more difficult, an overstretched back will also interfere with a patient's ability to do a functional lift (Figure 1–2). Much of the muscle power used will be wasted on elongating the stretched back rather than being used to lift the buttocks.

d. Rolling may be more difficult with an overstretched back and trunk. The shoulders will have to be brought over much farther before the hips will follow. Again, much of the power in the roll is wasted on elongating the trunk rather than on pulling the hips over.

e. The posture created by the overstretched back may compromise respiration.

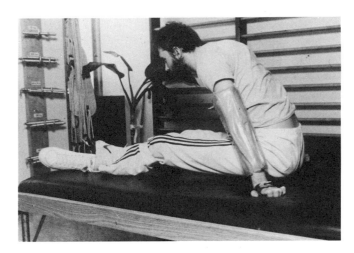

Figure 1–2 Overstretched upper back limits the ability to achieve a functional lift. Much of the patient's power is wasted on winging the scapula and elongating the overstretched back.

f. Selective tightness of the longer finger flexors will provide a functional grasp through a tenodesis motion.

g. Even if the patient will be dependent for most of his care, it will be easier to move and care for him if adequate ROM is maintained.

h. Pressure sore. The more easily the patient can move or be moved, the less likely it is that he will be in any one position long enough to develop pressure sores.

E. Muscle tone

1. Process to include:

    a. Description of *quantity* of tone

        (1) Mild increase. Resistance to passive stretch is noted but does not interfere with ROM or function.

        (2) Moderate increase. More resistance to passive stretch is noted. Full ROM is not prevented; however, tone may interfere with function (i.e., it may take longer to do transfers).

        (3) Severe increase. ROM will be impaired. Many functional skills are now impossible (i.e., patient may not be able to maintain long sitting even if placed in position).

    b. Description of *quality* of tone

        (1) Constant or fluctuating?

        (2) Does it occur with position changes?

(3) Is it symmetrical?

(4) Do fluctuations seem to be related to time of day?

(5) Can increased tone be used for functional activities?

c. Other considerations

(1) Recovery process. Spinal shock lasts three to six weeks. In upper motor neuron injuries, tone tends to increase for the first two years and then levels off. Flexor tone is usually more predominant initially; extensor tone may start increasing at six months.

(2) Medication

2. Implications for patient care:

a. ADL independence may be decreased or increased, depending on muscle tone present.

b. Depending on the quantity present, pressure sores may be more likely to occur because with increased tone:

(1) Good positioning can be more difficult.

(2) Any movement is generally harder.

(3) The skin may be pulled tighter, making bony prominences more prominent.

c. Other testing may be more difficult.

F. Strength (see Appendix F, Exhibit F–1)

1. Process to include:
Complete evaluation of all muscles

2. Difficulties to anticipate in testing:

a. Immobilization devices may interfere with proper positioning and thus accuracy. For instance, the SOMI usually restricts proper positioning in prone postures.

b. Stabilization of proximal joints and body parts is often impaired because of decreases in strength. A patient may have good to normal shoulder flexors but, because of poor trunk stabilization, appear to have only a fair muscle grade.

c. Substitutions are frequent; for example, a patient may use the rotator cuff and his position relative to gravity to straighten his elbow rather than triceps. Palpation is a must. (See Appendix B for frequent substitutions.)

d. Pain

3. Implications for patient care:

a. ADL independence. Strength is important in determining a patient's potential level of functional independence. Some key muscle groups and their functional significance are listed below:

(1) Scapular stabilizers—can facilitate a one-man pivot transfer and may make possible operation of an electric W/C with hand controls (scapular abduction and adduction are particularly important)

(2) Pectoralis major—necessary for rolling

(3) Biceps—used in bed mobility skills, in maintaining a stable sitting position in W/C (patient hooks arm behind push handle), and in assisting with transfer

(4) Wrist extensors—may be used to provide a functional grasp in absence of hand musculature (e.g., tenodesis), to assist with W/C propulsion, and to provide a ''hook'' to be used in other ADL (e.g., patient may hook his wrist under his knees and pull into sitting position)

(5) Triceps—presence makes performance of all ADL easier and less time consuming. A W/C push-up is now possible. Lateral transfers with and without a sliding board can be done with ease.

(6) Hip flexors—without this group, functional ambulation may not be possible.

(7) Knee flexors and extensors—ambulation will probably be functional and possible with use of AFOs. Less energy will be used in gait.

(8) Ankle dorsiflexors—ambulation will be possible with no assistive bracing.

b. Pressure sores. The more easily a patient can move or be moved, the less likely it is that he will be in any one position long enough to develop pressure sores.

G. Tolerance to vertical

1. Process to include:
Evaluation of vertical tolerance, which can be completed in bed, in a reclining W/C, or on a tilt table

2. Implications for patient care:

a. ADL independence. Decreased tolerance will affect transfers, W/C propulsion, dressing, and so on.

b. Admission may be extended.

c. Discharge plans may need to be altered, for example:

(1) Reclining W/Cs have a larger turning radius; this may create accessibility problems.

(2) If transfers are more difficult, an attendant may be required.

H. Balance

1. Process to include:
   a. Evaluation of presence of protective extension reaction
   b. Evaluation of presence of equilibrium reaction
   c. Evaluation of static balance versus dynamic balance
2. Implications for patient care:
   a. Unless patient has an accompanying head injury, deficits noted are usually the result of peripheral motor and sensory losses. Patient usually knows when he is falling; however, muscles he would ordinarily use to correct this are not working. Thus, he has to learn to substitute new muscles and movement patterns.
   b. Trunk supports may be needed to assist with balance.
   c. Because of the patient's need to stabilize with one hand, he may need to develop more skills with one-handed activities. Two-handed activities may no longer be as much of an option.

I. Coordination

1. Process to include:
   a. Evaluation of kinesthetic awareness (body sense), timing, and accuracy of movement
   b. Review of coordination skills prior to injury
2. Implications for patient care:
   a. Increased repetition may be needed for learning.
   b. Increased instruction, explanation, and verbal cues may facilitate learning a new task.
   c. Admission may be extended.
   d. Potential for ADL independence may be decreased.

J. Endurance

1. Process to include:
   a. Evaluation of cardiopulmonary status
   b. Evaluation of ability to coordinate good breathing patterns with activities
2. Implications for patient care:
   a. Patient may be physically able to do various ADL but unable to complete activity within a reasonable time period because of decreased endurance.
   b. Training may require more time because of the need for more rest periods and shorter exercise sessions.

K. ADL

1. Process to include:
   Evaluation of skills in areas of bed mobility, pressure relief, transfers, W/C mobility, and ambulation (see Appendix F, Exhibit F–2)
2. Implication for patient care:
   Discharge plans will vary depending on the level of independence achieved.

L. Problem-solving abilities

1. Process to include:
   a. Evaluation of patient's ability to solve problems independently. Does he need step-by-step explanations or just major guideposts?
   b. Evaluation of quality. Are his judgments and plans for approaching a situation safe?
   c. Evaluation of time needed to solve problems
2. Implications for patient care:
   a. Potential for ADL independence may be decreased.
   b. Discharge plans may be altered, depending on level of independence.

M. Affective components

1. Process to include:
   a. Evaluation of patient's understanding of his disability. Is he realistic?
   b. Evaluation of his acceptance of responsibility. Does he attend scheduled appointments? Does he use his problem-solving skills? Does he participate in equipment purchase decisions?
   c. Evaluation of his emotional status
2. Implications for patient care:
   a. Training may be delayed to accommodate affective components.

b. Potential for ADL independence may be decreased.

c. Discharge plans may be altered, depending on level of independence.

II. RELEVANT CHART INFORMATION

A. Onset of injury

Implications for patient care:
1. May aid in interpretation of affective components of behavior
2. May help define prognosis and thus goals. Is there potential for increased spasticity? Is there potential for increased return?
3. May indicate need to explore possible secondary medical complications, such as osteoporosis.

B. Type of injury (e.g., fracture dislocation, complete cord transection, tumor, hemisection, gunshot wound)

Implications for patient care:
1. May help define prognosis and thus goals
2. May help anticipate possible medical complications

C. General health status (e.g., head injury, other fractures, respiratory problems, cardiac problems, ectopic bone formation [see Appendix C], bowel and bladder problems)

Implications for patient care:
1. ADL independence may be limited. For example:
   a. Ectopic bone will cause decreases in ROM. Will this interfere with transfers?
   b. Cardiac and respiratory problems will probably affect endurance. If patient needs frequent rest periods, training may take longer. In addition, ultimate functional independence may be limited by decreased endurance.
2. Longer admission may be indicated.
3. Postures available for therapy may be restricted. For example:
   a. Ectopic bone may decrease ROM and make assumption of prone posture impossible.
   b. Respiratory problems may interfere with the use of prone posture.

D. Age

Implication for patient care:
ADL independence. Younger patients may be able to do more than older patients or be more adaptive to change.

E. Body build (Height, weight, proportions)

1. Present and premorbid weight should be considered. Patient usually returns to at least his original weight.
2. Implications for patient care:
   a. Pressure sores. A thin patient has more prominent bony areas and may be more prone to skin problems; however, a heavy patient may be difficult to move and thus is moved less often, creating an increased vulnerability to pressure areas.
   b. Discharge plans. For example:
      1. Equipment. Custom-built W/Cs have longer delivery times and often create added accessibility problems. Raised seats do not always fit under tables. Oversized W/Cs cannot fit through doors and may require a longer turning radius.
      2. Attendant care. A heavier patient may be less independent and require more people to assist with daily care. Will his family be able to do this? Is an attendant needed? Is an institutional setting indicated?

F. Premorbid personality and life style

1. Some considerations:
   a. Was personality rigid and unchanging, or was it more flexible?
   b. Did patient take responsibility for himself and his actions?
   c. Was he athletic or sedentary?
   d. What was his education level?
   e. What kind of job did he have?
2. Implications for patient care:
   a. Goals should be tailored to patient's life style (not the therapist's).
   b. A patient with a rigid personality may have difficulty seeing options in alternative life styles; therefore, he may be unable to attain

the ADL independence he is physically capable of achieving.

G. Family background

1. Some considerations:
   a. What is the educational history?
   b. What are the vocational demands?
   c. Are other health problems present in the family?
   d. Is the family supportive?
2. Implication for patient care:
   Discharge plans. Will the patient be discharged to home? If so, will special family training be needed? What equipment should be ordered? (The economic situation will influence decisions.)

H. Discharge plans

Implication for patient care:
If indicated in the charts, discharge plans can provide a starting point for goal setting and give some idea of the patient, family, and/or physician's expectations.

SUMMARY

Evaluation is a continuous process. Quality patient care includes not only an *initial* evaluation to collect baseline information and identify patient problems but also *interim* evaluations to determine whether the actual results are building toward the intended outcomes and *final* evaluations to determine whether the outcomes were achieved and to refine discharge plans.

General Outcomes

Goals are set after the initial evaluation is completed. However, goals are not just "set" one time. Patient care is a dynamic process. The therapist must continuously interpret new information, new observations, and the impact of programs conducted by himself and other team members. Therefore, goals are constantly being reevaluated and changed to meet the patient's needs.

This chapter deals with outcomes that all patients should be expected to meet, regardless of level of injury. In later units specific expectations for patients in relation to the level of injury will be discussed.

Outcome	*Considerations*	*Process*
1. Patient achieves maximum strength possible in all muscle groups.	1. Substitutions of stronger muscle groups may mask performance of weaker muscles. 2. Accurate evaluations and aggressive strengthening programs may be limited by: • ROM deficits • abnormal tone • immobilization devices • pressure sores, which may require special positioning	1. Evaluate muscle strength throughout. 2. Develop and implement exercise program to achieve the outcome with both resisted exercises and resisted functional activity, using all possible treatment settings and methods of facilitation: • mat programs • exercise classes • pool • independent work time • use of slings, pulleys, weights, powder boards, swiss ball, and so on. 3. Integrate program with other team members. 4. Provide a home program as indicated. 5. Evaluate patient and/or family performance of home program. 6. Periodically reevaluate muscle strength. 7. Upgrade home program as indicated.

Outcome	*Considerations*	*Process*
2. Patient maintains full ROM in all joints.	1. Limiting factors may include: • ectopic bone formations • abnormal tone • pain 2. Presence of pressure sores, which may require positioning that encourages contractures and/or makes ROM more difficult. 3. Ability of attendant or significant other to provide adequate ROM.	1. Evaluate passive ROM throughout; consider both osteokinematics and arthrokinematics. 2. Perform joint mobilization and passive ROM as indicated. 3. Consult OT to establish need for splinting and/or casting to assist with range. 4. Instruct patient to direct performance of ROM, and evaluate his ability to do this. 5. When indicated, provide both written and verbal instruction of ROM to other team members and significant other. 6. Instruct patient in self-ROM as indicated. 7. Evaluate patient's performance of self-ROM. Make corrections as needed. 8. Teach and evaluate positioning in bed and W/C to avoid contractures (e.g., prone lying, symmetrical posture in W/C). 9. Evaluate and provide equipment needed for proper positioning (e.g., appropriate foot supports, trunk supports). 10. Make appropriate adjustments on equipment to ensure good positioning. 11. Periodically reevaluate ROM, upgrading program as needed.

---

3. Patient attains maximum respiration capacity. *Components* a. Ability to maintain good bronchial hygiene: • mobilize secretions • clear secretions from lungs b. Respiratory skills maximally coordinated with all functional activities: • bed mobility • pressure relief • transfers • W/C mobility • ambulation • speech	1. Previous and current respiratory status: • allergies, asthma • respiratory complications related to injury • tracheostomy 2. Presence of pressure sores, abnormal tone, decreased ROM, and/or patient's general fear or discomfort with movement may make positioning and handling more difficult and may therefore limit attaining maximum respiratory capacity. 3. Equipment: What is available to assist? • abdominal binders (may increase VC and assist with coughing) • motorized reclining W/C may be considered to assist with position changes in sitting (which may decrease the potential for secretion pooling) 4. GPB may add as much as 1000 cc to patient's VC.	1. Evaluate present respiratory status and skills. 2. Improve ROM and strength of trunk and respiratory apparatus: • proximal joint ROM • chest expansion via airshifts, rotational exercises, and so on • strength of diaphragm and accessory muscles 3. Improve VC by: • positioning • creating good trunk stability (consider trunk supports) • improving breathing patterns • teaching GPB • using pool, respiratory classes, individual sessions 4. Teach skills to improve and/or maintain good bronchial hygiene: • Improve patient's comfort with being moved into as many different positions as possible.

Outcome	*Considerations*	*Process*
		• Teach coughing techniques.
		• Teach suctioning as indicated.
		• Teach postural drainage as indicated.
		5. Coordinate improved respiratory skills with functional activities:
		• speech (in conjunction with speech therapist)
		• improved endurance with ADL
		6. Incorporate skills into patient's daily routine.
		7. Evaluate performance during pass on nursing floor.
		8. Assist patient in problem solving to alleviate difficulties.
4. Patient maintains intact skin, free of pressure sores and other injury.	1. Presence of ectopic bone, abnormal tone, or pain may make positioning more difficult.	1. Evaluate sensation to determine sensory level.
	2. Fragile skin or existing lesions may require special procedures.	2. Issue interim equipment and order definitive W/C, seat cushion, and other equipment appropriate to pressure relief needs. (Inflated ring cushions can cause damage due to insufficient pressure distribution.)
	3. Some methods of transfer can provide more stress to skin than others.	3. Teach patient and/or significant other proper skin care procedures:
		• rolling to allow for position changes in bed
		• W/C pressure relief or push-ups
		• safety precautions during functional activities to prevent:
		• blunt force injuries (avoiding dropping legs, bouncing on buttocks, bumping, or crushing body parts, such as toes)
		• friction injuries on sheets and sliding boards and also on rough materials in transfers
		• thermal injuries (avoiding hot pipes and heaters and carrying hot objects and liquids in W/C; providing adequate clothing for extremities in cold weather)
		• pressure injuries (avoiding clothing constriction in groin, thick seams, tight shoes, putting items in back pants pockets, tightness of leg bag strap, and improper position of leg bag metal clamps)
		• moisture damage (changing damp clothing, ordering appropriate cushion for aeration)
		• appropriate positioning for care of skin or existing pressure sores

Outcome	Considerations	Process
		• proper adjustment of footrest for appropriate weight distribution over ischial tuberosities and thighs
		• awareness of proper cushion volume for pressure relief and maintenance procedures, if special cushion is ordered
		4. Evaluate performance of skin care procedures during daily routine.
		5. Assist patient in problem solving to alleviate difficulties.
5. Patient tolerates the vertical position symptom free.	1. Some medical problems may prevent vertical tolerance: • ectopic bone in hips • skin lesions • spinal instability	1. Issue abdominal binders and reclining W/C. 2. In conjunction with nursing program, gradually increase to vertical in a reclining W/C with elevating legrests. 3. Incorporate vertical positions in exercise program, especially work in long sitting. 4. Progress to a standard upright W/C when patient is able to tolerate the vertical position.
6. Patient attains maximum sitting tolerance (seven to eight hours if possible)	1. Existing lesions or fragile skin over superficial bony prominences may delay increases in sitting time. 2. Sitting tolerance may vary, depending on: • W/C prescription • type of cushion • method of pressure relief • availability of attendant or significant other to assist with relief	1. Evaluate motor components. 2. Determine realistic method of pressure relief. 3. Provide appropriate W/C and seat cushion for individual skin needs. 4. Instruct patient in pressure relief techniques. 5. Evaluate practice of pressure relief by patient or his direction of significant other's performance of pressure relief. 6. Increase sitting time in conjunction with nursing program. 7. Incorporate sitting time into other therapies.
7. Patient uses or compensates for abnormal tone. *Components* a. Compensation for both spasticity and flaccidity b. Use of or compensation for abnormal tone in all ADL: • bed mobility • pressure relief • transfers • W/C mobility • ambulation	1. Deficits in ROM and strength may limit compensatory techniques available to patient. 2. Poor body sense and coordination may interfere with patient's ability to learn compensatory techniques. 3. Increases in spasticity can be a warning signal for other medical complications, such as: • bowel and bladder distention • urinary tract infections and other septic conditions • local skin lesions, ingrowing toenails These should be ruled out before a treatment course is decided on.	1. Evaluate tone: • What kind is present? • How much? • Where is it located? • When does it occur? • Does it fluctuate? • Does time of day affect it? • Are fluctuations related to medication? • Where is patient in the recovery process? 2. Teach patient and/or significant other to recognize limitations imposed by abnormal tone.

Outcome	*Considerations*	*Process*
		3. If indicated, teach patient and significant other techniques to reduce spasticity:
		• ROM
		• prolonged stretch (e.g., sleeping in a prone position may reduce flexor tone; lying supine with legs in a tailor position may decrease lower extremity extensor tone)
		• postures that eliminate the pull of gravity on spastic muscles
		• FES (see Appendix D)
		• joint mobilization
		• heat and cold modalities, weight-bearing activities, rhythmic rotational movements, and so on
		4. Teach patient to use and/or compensate for abnormal tone.
		5. Incorporate skills into patient's daily routine on nursing floor, in other therapies, and on passes.
		6. Assist patient and significant other in problem solving to alleviate difficulties.
8. Patient achieves maximum cardiovascular endurance. *Components* Maximum endurance to be achieved in: • all ADL (including bed mobility, transfers, W/C mobility, ambulation) • all exercise	1. Limiting factors may include: • other medical problems • age • obesity	1. Evaluate respiratory skills and cardiac response. 2. Improve respiratory skills. 3. Incorporate respiratory skills into ADL and daily routine. 4. Grade exercise and activity to increase endurance. 5. Monitor heart rate and blood pressure as indicated. 6. Teach patient how to grade his exercise and activity to increase endurance.
9. Patient achieves maximum sitting balance. *Components* a. Long and short sitting balance: • with bilateral upper extremity support • with unilateral upper extremity support • without upper extremity support b. Sitting balance within: • W/C • car • tub and toilet, if indicated	1. Available strength may determine method used. 2. ROM: Normal ROM is particularly important at the hips and elbows. 3. Muscle length (both tightness and excessive length), especially to be considered: • hamstrings (should be no greater than 110 degrees) • low back musculature 4. Tone 5. Coordination (patient's ability to learn new movement patterns)	1. Evaluate motor components. 2. Evaluate functional component parts found in developmental postures: • head control • weight shifting ability • protective extension reactions • equilibrium responses • ability to find one's COG • compensatory sensory techniques 3. Teach functional component parts in lower postures. 4. Improve motor components such as ROM, strength, tolerance to vertical, and so on.

Outcome	*Considerations*	*Process*
	6. Tolerance to vertical	5. Teach sitting balance.
	7. Patient's fear of falling may slow training.	6. Progress from long sitting (larger base of support, thus more stable) to short sitting.
		7. Progress from bilateral upper extremity support to unilateral support to without upper extremity support.
		8. Include use of any and all facilitatory techniques.
		9. Include use of any and all equipment and teaching settings (e.g., mats, pool, pulleys, weights, swiss ball, slings)
		10. Progress to using sitting balance with functional activities (e.g., ball games, wheeling W/C)

---

10. Patient achieves maximum independence with bed mobility activities.	1. Strength	1. Evaluate motor skills present.
	2. ROM: Full ROM is particularly important at shoulders and hips.	2. Evaluate functional component skills found in developmental postures.
Components	3. Tone	3. Evaluate potential equipment needs.
a. Rolling to right and left	4. What immobilization devices are used? These can make the activity more difficult.	4. Improve motor skills.
b. Rolling from prone to supine and back		5. Teach functional component skills in various postures through exercise progression considering all methods of facilitation and all possible treatment modalities.
c. Moving from supine to sitting (both long sitting and short sitting) and return to supine	5. Pressure sores and fragile skin (may make activities more difficult)	
d. Moving to either side of the bed	6. Equipment: What is available to assist?	6. Teach bed mobility skills.
e. Moving to head and foot of the bed	• bed (manual, electric)	7. Practice activities in part and whole.
f. Performing pressure relief in bed	• controls used on bed	8. Teach skills on mat first (firmer surface); then progress to bed.
	• mattress (softer mattresses make movement more difficult)	9. Prescribe equipment.
		10. Instruct nursing staff, OT, and significant other in patient's bed mobility patterns.
		11. Incorporate skills into patient's daily routine on nursing floor and on passes.
		12. Evaluate performance on nursing floor and on passes.
		13. Assist patient and significant other in problem solving to alleviate difficulties.

---

11. W/C dependent patient demonstrates the ability to direct, assist with, or operate a W/C indoors and outdoors.	1. Strength	1. Evaluate motor skills present.
	2. ROM:	2. Evaluate functional component skills found in developmental postures.
Components	• operation of W/C easiest with at least 90 degrees of hip flexion.	3. Evaluate for appropriate W/C.
a. Forward–backward turns	• if using manual W/C, shoulder extension particularly important	4. Improve motor skills.
b. Safe fall out of W/C		

Outcome	*Considerations*	*Process*
c. Management of all W/C parts	3. Tone	5. Teach functional component skills in various postures through exercise progression considering all methods of facilitation and all possible treatment modalities.
d. Management of doors	4. Sensation	
e. Indoors:	5. Coordination	
• all surfaces, tile to carpet	6. Endurance	6. Create trunk stability in W/C via:
• doorways	7. Equipment: What is available to assist?	• increased sitting balance skills
• maneuvering in tight places	• type of W/C	• possible higher back to W/C
• elevators	• type of controls on W/C	• trunk supports, straps
• elevations	• W/C accessories (e.g., brake extensions, ramp retarders)	• cushion, solid seat inserts, and so on.
f. Outdoors:		7. Teach W/C skills, beginning with foward propulsion.
• all terrains		8. Progress: indoors to outdoors, smooth terrain to rough, wider areas to narrower, level to elevations.
• elevations (ramps, curbs, bumps, and cracks in sidewalk)		9. Develop problem-solving skills via outdoor trips and/or passes that cover various commonly encountered problems:
• crossing streets safely		• crowds
		• buildings that initially appear inaccessible
		• dealing with slanting sidewalks
		• bumps and cracks in sidewalks
		• other vehicles
		10. Increase endurance.
		11. Prescribe appropriate W/C.
		12. Instruct nursing staff, other team members, and significant other in patient's bed mobility patterns.
		13. Incorporate skills into patient's daily routine on nursing floor and on pass at home.
		14. Evaluate performance on nursing floor and on passes.
		15. Assist patient in problem solving to alleviate difficulties on nursing floor and at home.

12. Patient achieves maximum independence with transfers to all surfaces.	1. Strength	1. Evaluate motor skills present.
Components	2. ROM: Full ROM is particularly important at promixal joints.	2. Evaluate functional component skills found in developmental postures.
a. All aspects of transfer:	3. Pain	3. Assess potential architectural barriers and discharge plans.
• positioning of W/C	4. Tone	4. Evaluate for potential equipment needs.
• management of W/C parts	5. Sensation	5. Improve motor skills.
• management of equipment used to assist transfer	6. Endurance	6. Teach functional component skills in various postures through exercise progression considering all methods of facilitation and all possible treatment modalities.
• actual move from one surface to the next	7. Coordination	
• supine to sitting and back (including management of lower extremities)	8. Body build: weight, body proportions	
	9. Fear of falling	

Outcome	*Considerations*	*Process*
b. Transfer to all surfaces: • bed • bath • toilet • car • floor c. Emergency alternative transfer	10. Equipment: What is available to assist? • type of W/C • cushion • sliding board • bed mattress (usually easier on a firmer one) • type of car (two-door cars usually easier) 11. Toilet and bath transfers: • transfers more difficult when everything is wet • clothing	7. Teach transfer skills: • Break transfer down into component parts (e.g., position W/C, locking brakes, actual slide) • Practice transfer in part and whole. • Progress mat to bed to other transfers. • Progress from passive to active, assisted to independent. • Encourage patient to solve problems so that he has as much variety in approach as possible. 8. Teach emergency alternative transfer. 9. Prescribe equipment. 10. Instruct nursing staff, other team members, and significant other in patient's transfer patterns. 11. Incorporate skills into patient's daily routine on nursing floor and on pass at home. 12. Evaluate performance on nursing floor and on passes. 13. Assist patient in problem solving to alleviate difficulties on nursing floor and at home.
13. Ambulatory patients achieve maximum functional ambulation status. *Components* a. Donning and doffing orthosis b. Moving forward, backward, sideways, and turning to both right and left c. All surfaces—smooth to rough and uneven (e.g., sand, grass, carpets, tile) d. Maneuvering in narrow spaces e. Elevations: • stairs • ramps • curbs: two-inch, four-inch, and six-inch f. Elevators g. Escalators h. Standing to sitting to standing from all chairs i. Ability to fall safely j. Ability to assume standing from floor	1. Strength (most successful when at least some hip flexors present) 2. ROM: Most successful when: • hips have at least neutral extension • knees have full motion • ankles can achieve at least neutral dorsiflexion 3. Tone 4. Body weight: weight, body proportions • may be easier for thinner, shorter person 5. Endurance. Energy expenditure for this activity very high (two to four times greater than normal walking). 6. Motivation 7. Fear of falling 8. Equipment: What is available to assist? • type of orthosis • assistive devices	1. Evaluate motor skills present. 2. Evaluate functional component skills found in developmental postures. 3. Evaluate need for orthotic devices; consider consultation with orthotist. 4. Prescribe definitive orthosis as needed. 5. Improve motor skills. 6. Teach functional component skills in various postures through exercise progression considering all methods of facilitation and all possible treatment modalities. 7. Teach ambulatory skills: • Progress from parallel bars to assistive devices. • Develop forward progression, then proceed to backward, sideways, and turning. • Progress from smooth surfaces to rough, indoors to outdoors, level to elevations. • Increase endurance and speed. • Teach standing to sitting and back. • Teach controlled falling.

Outcome	Considerations	Process
		• Teach assumption of standing from floor.
		• Teach as many alternative gait patterns as possible.
		8. Instruct nursing staff, other team members, and significant other in patient's gait patterns.
		9. Incorporate skills into patient's daily routine in other therapies, on nursing floor, and on pass at home.
		10. Evaluate performance on nursing floor and on passes.
		11. Assist patient in problem solving to alleviate difficulties on nursing floor and at home.

---

14. Patient demonstrates awareness of proper operation and maintenance of equipment.

    Components

    All equipment prescribed by PT:

    • W/C
    • bath equipment
    • beds
    • orthosis
    • assistive gait devices
    • exercise equipment

1. Mentation, intellect
2. Mechanical abilities of patient
3. Sophistication of equipment prescribed
4. Availability of vendors, sources of repair, and rehabilitation facility to place of discharge

1. Evaluate mentation, intellect, and mechanical abilities.
2. Prescribe appropriate equipment.
3. Teach correct use of equipment and maintenance suggestions.
4. Teach common reasons for needing repair.
5. Teach how to repair simple problems.
6. Teach procedure for replacing damaged part.
7. Teach procedure for receiving repairs of equipment too difficult to handle by self (include list of vendors or sources for parts).
8. Include both written and verbal instructions as indicated.

---

15. Patient attains maximum mobility in home and community environment.

    Components

    a. Home
    b. Work
    c. Leisure settings
    d. All areas of community
    e. Mobility within designated setting and getting to and from setting

1. Patient acceptance of disability
2. Patient motivation
3. Support from significant other
4. Discharge plans
    • What will be the demands of his environment? Will he be discharged to a nursing home with tile floors and wide hallways, or will he live on a farm with uneven ground?
    • Will there be different demands at home as opposed to work or school?
    • Will W/C need to be transported?
    • What transportation is available to patient?
    • Will he have attendant care?

1. Evaluate functional independence.
2. Evaluate accessibility of discharge environment:
    • indoors
    • outdoors
    • work, school, leisure areas
3. Assist patient, significant others, and other team members in problem solving to eliminate architectural barriers.
4. Evaluate and prescribe appropriate equipment.
5. Refer to information sources:
    • recreation department
    • social work

Outcome	*Considerations*	*Process*
	5. Financial resources (What equipment can he afford?)	• local independent living centers
		• community referrals
		• Department of Rehabilitation Services
		• others
		6. Assist in planning passes.
		7. After pass, review weekend with significant other and patient; assist with problem solving to alleviate difficulties.

16. Significant other demonstrates ability to supervise and/or assist with all care and ADL as needed.
 	
Components
a. Respiratory care
b. ROM maintenance
c. Management of tone
d. Bed mobility
e. Transfers
f. Pressure relief
g. Maneuvering W/C in all settings
h. Equipment maintenance
i. Exercise programs
	1. Presence of spasticity, pain, contractures, and other medical complications
	
	2. Patient's body proportions, weight, height, and difficulty in moving
	
	3. Patient's ability to direct activity
	
	4. Significant other's:
	  • ability to learn new tasks
	  • physical and medical limitations
	  • ability to deal with psychological and role changes
	
	5. Discharge plans:
	  • Where
	  • How often will assist be needed? (All day, only on weekends, in evening?)
	  • How many people will be available to assist?
	  • Will there be architectural barriers?
	
	6. Equipment: What is available to assist? (Some equipment may facilitate better body mechanics and simplify care, such as an electric bed.)
		1. Assess discharge environment early, asking for home assessment form to be completed.
		
		2. Assess physical, emotional, and medical limitations of significant other.
		
		3. Note patient's size, height, weight, and body proportions.
		
		4. Determine appropriate procedures for various activities.
		
		5. Demonstrate activity to significant other.
		
		6. Observe significant other return-demonstrations (consider teaching him with able-bodied person first).
		
		7. Ask for several repetitions of activity to verify that significant other is comfortable and safe.
		
		8. Simulate discharge situations as much as possible.
		
		9. Arrange for significant other to practice activities on nursing floor.
		
		10. Notify team that patient is ready for pass.
		
		11. After pass, review weekend with significant other and patient, assisting with problem solving to alleviate difficulties.
		
		12. Observe demonstration of solutions.

17. Patient demonstrates the ability to direct all his care.
 	
Components
a. Respiratory care
b. ROM maintenance
c. Management of tone
d. Bed mobility
e. Transfers
	1. Patient personality prior to injury:
	  • How assertive was he?
	
	2. Respiratory status
	  • How well is it coordinated with speech? How many syllables can he say per breath? Is his voice volume impaired?
	  • Does he have a tracheostomy?
	  • Have vocal cords been damaged?
	
	3. Mental deficits
		1. Evaluate respiratory skills as they relate to speech.
		
		2. Evaluate mentation.
		
		3. Determine appropriate procedures for various activities.
		
		4. Practice various procedures with patient.
		
		5. Teach steps to accomplish each procedure, emphasizing good body mechanics and safety.

Outcome	*Considerations*	*Process*
f. Pressure relief		6. Instruct patient to direct PT with each activity.
g. Maneuvering W/C in all settings		7. Instruct patient to direct significant other and/or stranger.
h. Equipment maintenance		8. Instruct nursing staff in patient's movement patterns.
i. Exercise programs		9. Incorporate patient's direction of his care into his daily routine on nursing floor and at home on pass.
		10. Evaluate performance on nursing floor and on pass.
		11. Assist patient in problem solving to alleviate difficulties.

Developing a Treatment Plan

GENERAL TREATMENT PRINCIPLES

As is true in so many other areas of this treatment process, treatment planning principles for the SCI patient are no different than those underlying the treatment of patients with many other diagnoses and disabilities. Some of these are highlighted below:

- *Teaching a Process for Solving Problems:* Disabled persons will never be able to learn how to approach every obstacle they are likely to encounter in life during their rehabilitation stay. It is therefore important for the therapist to teach the patient how to solve problems.

  In the process of treatment a patient will learn many concrete tasks—how to roll, how to assume sitting, how to transfer into the bed, and so on. However, these concrete tasks should not be viewed as ends themselves, but rather as the means for teaching the patient how to solve problems.

  This means that while the therapist still needs to provide the patient with some success, he cannot give him all the answers. The patient should be allowed to exhaust his problem-solving skills first. Even at this point, a skilled therapist will be able to give the patient a few cues or perhaps the next step without giving him the whole answer. Like anything else, problem-solving skills need to be challenged in order for them to improve.

- *Going Through the Motion:* Patients, just like everyone else, learn skills by getting a "feel" for the movement. Able-bodied individuals are able to watch a movement and then grossly move through it on their own before breaking it down into its component parts for practice. The patient, on the other hand, is often only able to do this if the therapist assists him. Learning will be easier for the patient if the therapist will take time to do this. As the patient is assisted through the movement, he will be able to develop his own "feel" for the task and thus be more efficient in his practice of component parts, ultimately being able to learn the whole task more quickly.

- *Success:* Even at the beginning of treatment, the patient needs to be successful to ensure good motivation and carry-over. This can make finding an appropriate starting point a bit of a challenge. However, one key to determining a starting point can always be found by looking at the patient. For example, treatment programs for the patient with marked extensor tone may not begin with the patient in a supine position. This might only serve to accentuate the tone and frustrate the patient with his failure to perform the given task.

- *Working in Reverse:* Working forward through a progression is not always the most appropriate approach. Again, start where the patient will be most successful. What at first seems to be the more usual progression may not always meet the patient's needs. Working in reverse can often be a more successful experience. If it is easier for the patient to learn how to assume sitting starting from the sitting posture and working down to supine, do not insist that he start from supine and work his way forward to sitting.

- *Narrowing the Problem:* How a treatment program is actually structured will depend on the results of the evaluation and on the desired goals. However, general evaluations and questions will only point to a general direction. For example, an MMT will only give a general idea of weakness. The problem needs to be narrowed before adequate strengthening programs can be developed. In order to do this more specific questions need to be asked.

What is actually causing the weakness—partial innervation of the muscle or increases in tone? If increased tone is a factor, relaxation techniques will need to be incorporated into the program.

Why does the patient need to be stronger? What activity is the strength needed for? Unless treatment programs are meaningful, maintaining patient interest and motivation will be difficult.

Strengthening programs will always have better carry-over if muscles are strengthened in the way in which they will be used functionally. This knowledge leads to further questions.

In what part of the range does the patient need more strength? Is the strength needed in the shortened end of the range, as is the case with the pectoralis major if it is to assist in maintaining the prone-on-elbow posture, or is it needed in the lengthened end of the range, as is the case with the anterior deltoid muscles if they are to assist in W/C propulsion.

What type of muscle contraction will be used in the activity—isometric or isotonic, concentric, or eccentric? How will the muscle be used in the activity? Will it be used in isolation, as the pectoralis muscles are often used to accomplish elbow locking in the absence of triceps, or will it be used in combination with other muscle groups, as the C6-quadriplegic frequently combines the deltoids and forearm pronators to push a W/C? Perhaps the muscle will even be used as part of a substitution pattern. For example, the C5-quadriplegic, when feeding, often needs to use the internal shoulder rotators to substitute for poor forearm pronators.

Does the patient need more endurance or power to accomplish the activity? If endurance is the goal, resistance will be decreased while the number of repetitions required is increased. If muscle power is the goal, the reverse is true. Resistance will be increased, but the number of repetitions will be decreased.

- *Developing a Balance of Skills:* Much of the patient's success in accomplishing a task is found in a balance between motor skills. Because of this, treatment programs need to be developed with a consciousness of both what a patient will gain and what he will lose from a skill. Excessive ROM may facilitate better body mechanics in some situations, but it may also mean that the patient will need to develop more power, either through increased muscle strength or skilled use of momentum, to accomplish other tasks.

For example, to accomplish a roll, the patient with a very flexible trunk will have to be able to bring his shoulders much farther past the midline before his hips will follow than the patient with a tighter trunk. The patient who is able to bring his head to his knees in a long sitting position may be better able to shift his weight forward off his buttocks for a transfer but may be completely unable to develop enough power to regain and/or maintain a stable position in sitting without support.

This is not to say that there is an absolute right amount of ROM that each patient should strive for. Each patient will start at a different point and therefore have different end points. Some will naturally have more flexibility or more tightness than others.

No one motor skill can be developed in isolation from the others. Each patient will develop his own special blend of skills. It is this blend of skills that provides functional success, and this is one reason why there are so many different approaches to the same task. Therefore, the patient who seems to have a particular flair for using body mechanics to move should possibly be encouraged to develop more flexibility and ROM. However, this may not be the case for the patient who appears to have more difficulty grasping this concept of movement. His program may need to emphasize increased muscle tightness and strength.

Compromises are always being made. If both the patient and the therapist are aware of this from the beginning, treatment programs will be more relevant and efficient and the patient may achieve greater functional and physical independence in a shorter period of time.

- *Organizing the Treatment Plan:* The treatment plan is organized around two axes—the use of various postures within the developmental sequence and the stages of motor control (mobility, stability, controlled mobility skill). Exercises are done in progression using various positions in the developmental sequence: prone-on-elbows, supine-on-elbows, sidelying, hands and knees, sitting, kneeling, and standing. Activities from the second axis—the stages of motor control—are then superimposed upon these postures. Each sequence begins with an activity that provides the patient enough *mobility* to assume or be placed in the posture and advances through to activities that promote *stability, controlled mobility* (e.g., weight shifting where there is proximal movement over fixed distal parts), and, finally, *skill* in functional use (proximal parts are now fixed while distal parts move).

  Constant evaluation and reevaluation are needed to determine at which level of control the patient should be working in each posture. At any stage in treatment, the patient should be working in several postures using activities from the appropriate stage of control. The patient should always be maximally challenged, progressing to the highest level possible in each sequence.

  These progressions of motor control within the developmental sequence are the cornerstone of the treatment program for the SCI patient in that they combine many of the short-term goals with functional training. While advancing through the exercise sequences, the patient gains strength and functional ROM, learns functional patterns of movement (such as how to use his arms and upper trunk to move his lower trunk and legs), becomes aware of balance points and the position of his body in space, gains improved cardiopulmonary endurance, and solves problems to discover the most efficient method of accomplishing functional tasks.

- *Variety:* Often these progressions are done in the form of mat activities. However, class therapy, pool therapy, and the use of equipment, such as sling suspension, wall pulleys, equilibrium boards and so on, may be used to supplement and complement the basic mat exercise program. Everyone, including patients, becomes bored doing the same thing day after day. Treatment programs must have variety to maintain patient interest and motivation.

For example, *sling suspension* can be useful when trying to strengthen muscles with grades less than fair and when assistance is needed to support an extremity. Sling suspension is one way to offer the patient an opportunity to work independently on repetitions and requires only an occasional change in set-ups by a therapist or an aide.

Pool programs can also be used to augment strengthening programs as well as general mobility exercise programs. Water is an excellent medium owing to its buoyance and resistance properties to provide assistive and resistive exercise. To decrease patient fear, a jacket can be used, and, if necessary, wrist or ankle flotation devices can be used for support of limbs.

Programs can be implemented to meet individual goals. It is possible to work on breathing exercises. Balance in short sitting positions and rolling mobility can be initiated in the pool. Gait can be started in parallel bars in the pool when appropriate. Creative use of equipment, water games, and swimming strokes to achieve muscle strengthening, coordination, balance, and improved endurance are all valuable in the rehabilitation process. An example of a therapeutic pool record is presented in Appendix F, Exhibit F–6.

Note: Pool activity is contraindicated for anyone with open lesions, bowel or bladder incontinence (unless a catheter is used), allergic reactions to chlorine, isolation precautions, and spinal instability unless an orthosis can be worn in the pool.

Class programs provide an excellent forum for group exercise, interaction, competition, and repetition and are economical in use of staff time. Individual sessions can then be devoted to individual needs in mat programs and ADL development. See Appendix E for specific class information and Appendix F, Exhibit F–5 for an example of an exercise class form.

Several classes are appropriate for the patient with SCI:

- Classes in advanced upper extremity strengthening emphasize upper extremity and trunk strengthening using resistance, balance exercise, respiratory exercises, mobility, and endurance training.
- Beginning and intermediate upper extremity strengthening classes are designed for the patient with quadriplegia who uses little or no resistance

to exercise or can only exercise against gravity to a limited extent.

- Sling suspension classes can be used to offer support in gravity-eliminated positions for upper and lower extremities.
- W/C mobility skills classes can be used to build endurance and work on elevation skills, such as wheelies and curb jumping and ramps, and stairs negotiation as well as on other skills to be tried indoors or outdoors.
- Lower extremity strengthening classes emphasize strengthening of the lower extremities and trunk.

Classes should be distinguished from group activity in that they should be conducted using classroom techniques in the selection, organization, and implementation of a program that varies as the population changes. Primary therapists are responsible for giving input and monitoring the progression of their patients in the class. But the class therapist is responsible for providing activities that vary from day to day and for including a variety of exercises or activities on a mat or in a W/C

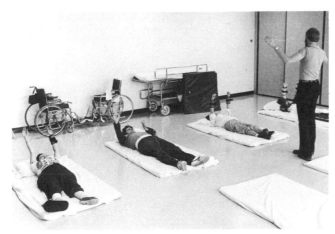

Figure 3–1 Exercises to develop strength can be performed in a class setting.

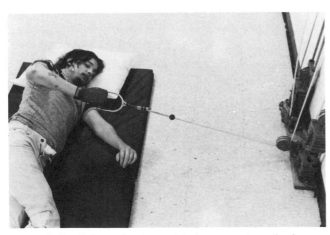

Figure 3–2a Pulley setup is used to increase strength of upper extremity.

designed to achieve strengthening and functional goals specific to the needs of the current patient population.

The addition of class and pool programs as well as the use of equipment lends variety to the treatment program, heightens motivation, and extends work periods, thus hastening development of maximal functional independence. A creative therapist will be able to use these activities to progress the patient through all levels of motor control.

TREATMENT OPTIONS

The following pages include a more specific discussion of the various stages of motor control as well as some examples of activities that might be used in treatment. What might be considered the more traditional mat progressions are not shown. This is not because they no longer have a place in treatment; they are, in fact, the mainstay of most SCI treatment programs. However, many sources have already well illustrated these progressions, notably P.E. Sullivan in her book *An Integrated Approach to Therapeutic Exercise: Theory and Clinical Practice*. Several other sources are also listed in the bibliography.

Again, this is not meant to be a cookbook of ideas. The intent is only to illustrate the process and show how equipment might be used to guide a patient through the levels of motor control in various developmental postures.

Mobility

This level of control will provide the prerequisites needed to progress through the next three stages. It will provide the motor skills, such as ROM and strength, that are needed to assume the various developmental postures. Examples of exercise to develop mobility are shown in Figures 3–1 through 3–3f.

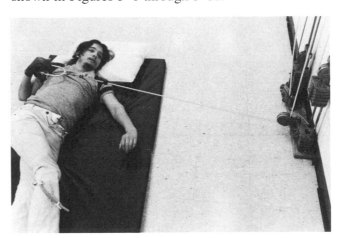

Figure 3–2b

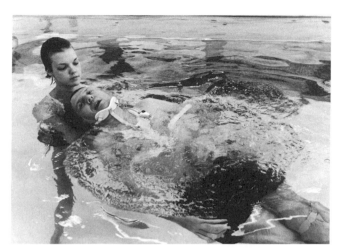

Figure 3–3a Exercises done in a pool help to develop trunk flexibility and upper extremity strength.

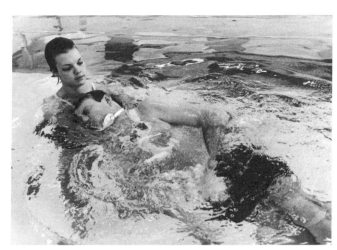

Figure 3–3b

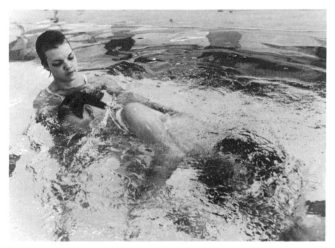

Figure 3–3c

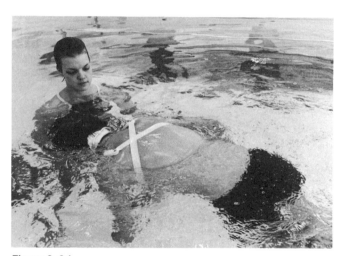

Figure 3–3d

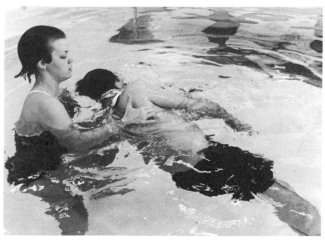

Figure 3–3e

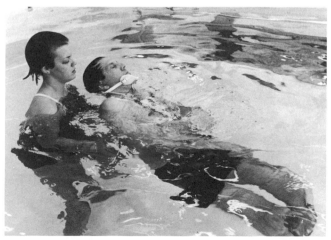

Figure 3–3f

Equipment can be used not only to develop these skills but also to assist a patient into a posture before these skills are fully developed (Figures 3–4 through 3–6b).

Stability

At this stage, the patient is learning static balance. The question is: when should activities begin to focus on this level of control? For example, if a patient does not have enough mobility (e.g., ROM in shoulder

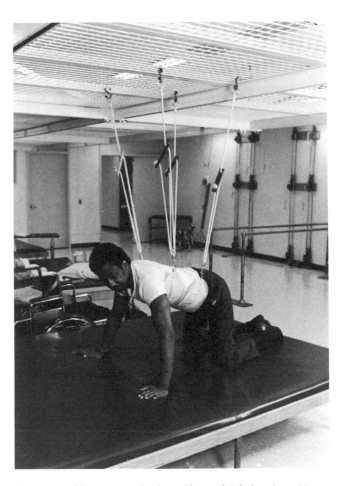

Figure 3–5 Sling suspension is used to maintain hands and knees position.

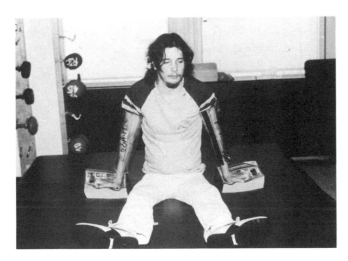

Figure 3–4 Air splints are used to maintain elbow extension.

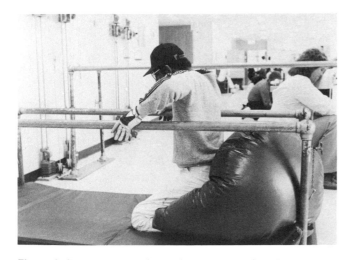

Figure 3–6a Bean bag assists patient to assume kneeling position.

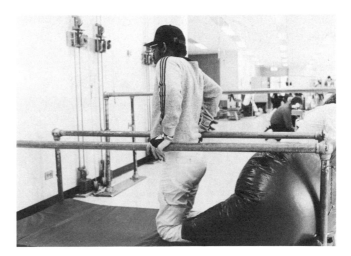

Figure 3–6b

extension) to achieve a supine-on-elbows posture, should the posture be used to develop stability?

Some believe that if this position is not pushed early, the patient may never be comfortable in it. So a little pain at the shoulders now is worth it. He will eventually stretch into shoulder extension and will then have many more functional options available to him to use as he learns to assume higher postures.

But what if the pain does not go away? Is the supine-on-elbows position that important? It may not be with some patients. They may be able to use other starting positions just as effectively to assume higher postures. If this is the case, perhaps the supine-on-elbows position should be avoided until enough mobility is present. Long sitting with upper extremity support might be a better position in which to develop stability. Even though the patient has the additional elbow joint to stabilize, this posture requires less shoulder extension.

Examples of activities to promote stability are shown in Figures 3–7 through 3–10.

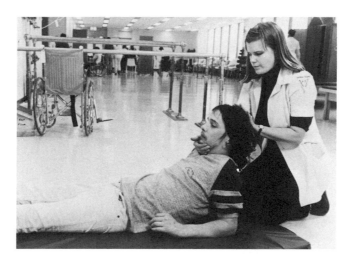

Figure 3–7 Resistance is applied through to head to encourage shoulder stabilization.

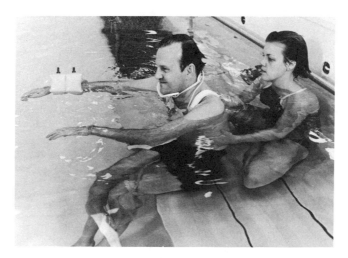

Figure 3–8 The resistance of the water is used to promote trunk stability.

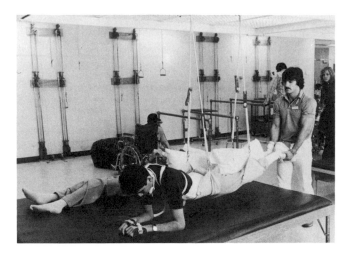

Figure 3–9 With the use of a sling setup resistance is applied through the feet to promote stability at the shoulders.

Controlled Mobility

This level of control develops dynamic balance. The distal parts are fixed while the proximal parts move. The patient develops kinesthetic awareness and the ability to move in and out of his base of support. He can now experiment with the speed and velocity of movement. Activities to develop dynamic balance and to control movement are shown in Figures 3–11a through 3–16.

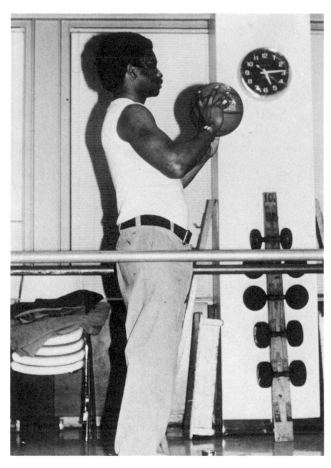

Figure 3–10 Stability is encouraged at the hip through the use of a skilled activity performed by the upper extremities.

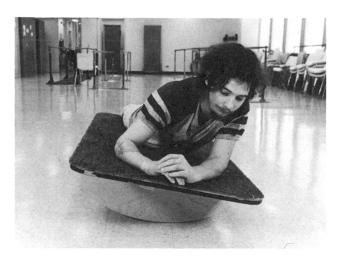

Figure 3–11a Patient uses rocker board to challenge dynamic balance.

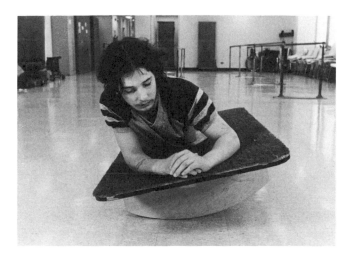

Figure 3–11b

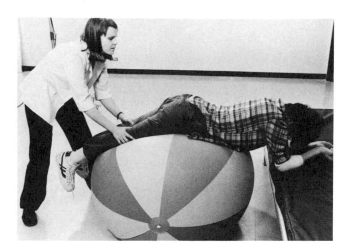

Figure 3–12a Patient is learning to control movement of his lower trunk through his upper extremities. He pushes the Bobath ball away, pulls it back to the table, and then moves his hips from side to side. This is an easy and fun activity to do with children, but a little more difficult to do with adults. Two people are usually required for the initial positioning on the ball.

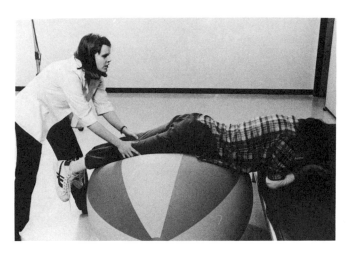

Figure 3–12b

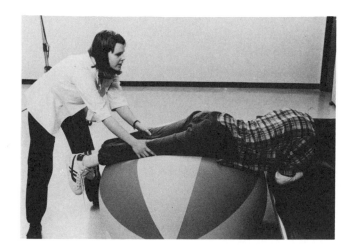

Figure 3–12c

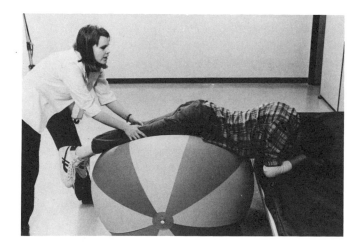

Figure 3–12d

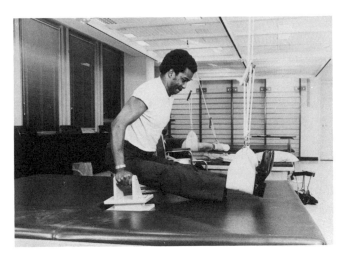

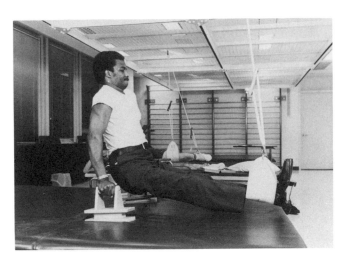

Figure 3–13a A sling suspension setup is used in combination with push-up blocks to develop controlled mobility. Note the use of scapular depressors, latissimus dorsi, hip hikers, and abdominal muscle groups.

Figure 3–13b

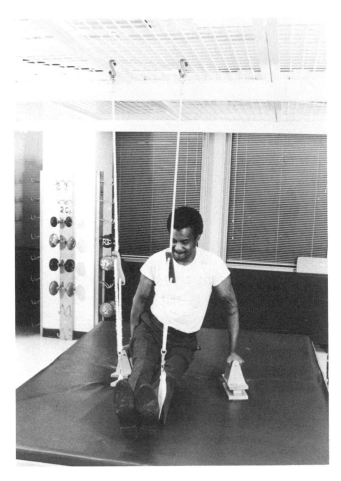

Figure 3–13c

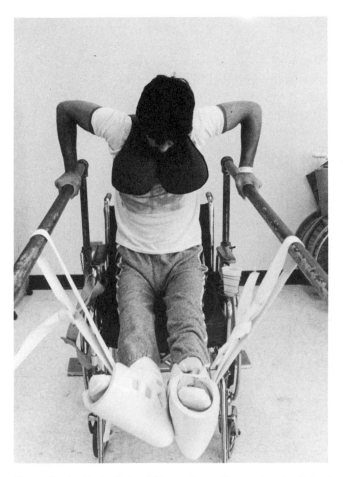

Figure 3–14a Controlled mobility in a long sitting posture is attained with a strap across the bars and weights on the shoulders to add resistance.

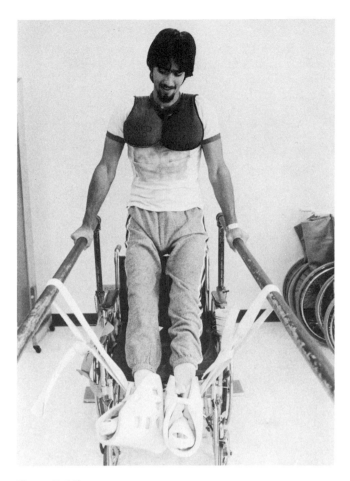

Figure 3–14b

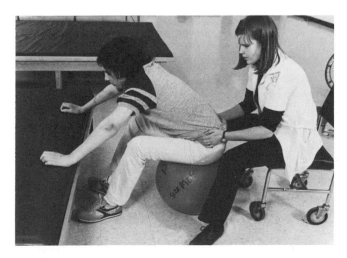

Figure 3–15a Patient is asked to push the Swiss ball away from the table and then pull it back in. Side to side as well as bouncing activities can be included.

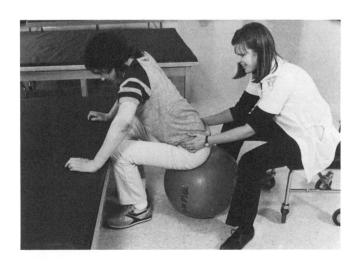

Figure 3–15b

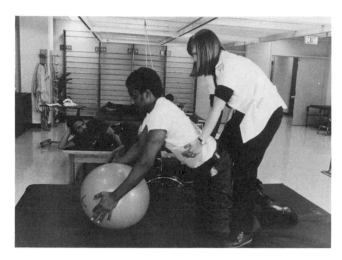

Figure 3–16 Kneeling patient is rolling the ball in as many directions as possible.

Static-Dynamic Activities

Many patients have difficulty moving directly from controlled mobility to the skill level. Static-dynamic activities provide a transition (Figures 3–17a through 3–19). One extremity will maintain a fixed distal component while the other experiments with proximal stabilization and distal movement.

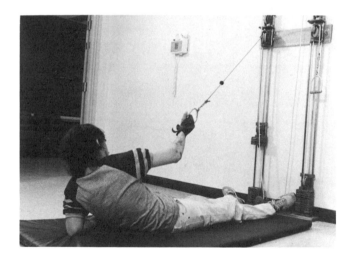

Figure 3–17a Patient performs a static-dynamic activity using pulleys in a supine-on-elbows position.

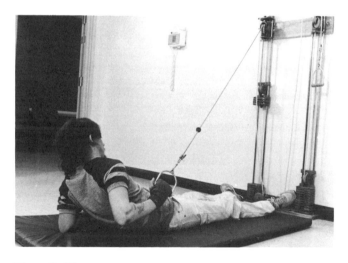

Figure 3–17b

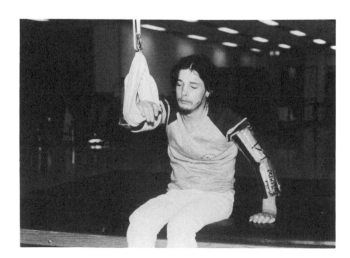

Figure 3–18a Patient is performing a static-dynamic activity using air splints and sling suspension.

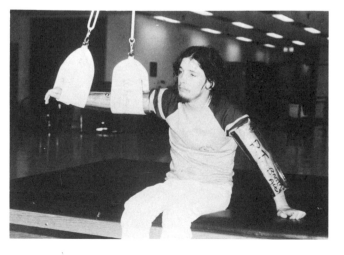

Figure 3–18b

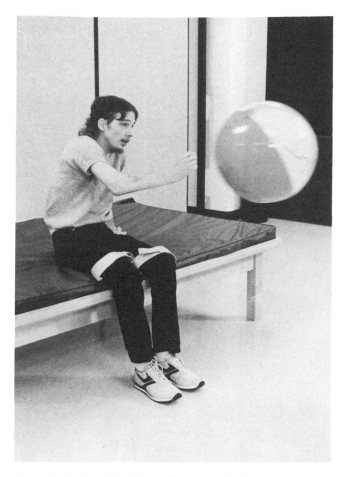

Figure 3–19 A beach ball is used by a patient in short sitting position to develop static-dynamic control.

Skill

At this final level of control proximal parts are now fixed while the distal parts move. Most functional activities require varying degrees of this level of control. Various exercises to develop skill are shown in Figures 3–20a through 3–23.

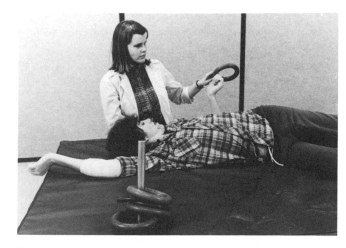

Figure 3–20a Rings are used to develop skill in sidelying.

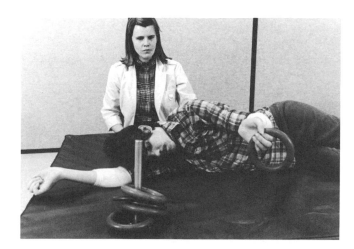

Figure 3–20b

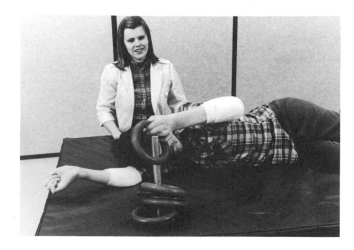

Figure 3–20c

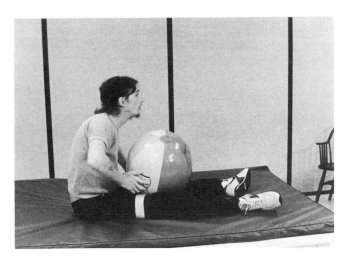

Figure 3–21a Playing catch with a beach ball can develop skill in long sitting.

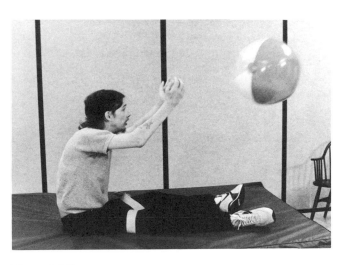

Figure 3–21b

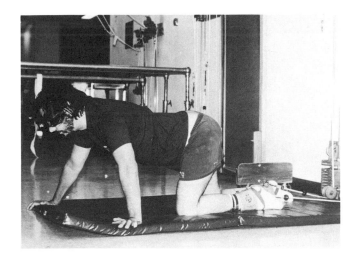

Figure 3–22 Skill can be attained in a hands and knees position by using pulleys.

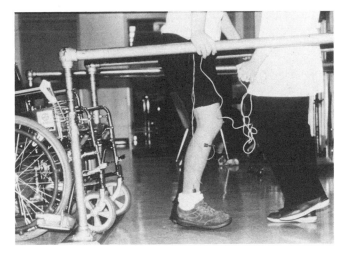

Figure 3–23 FES can be used to develop skill with walking. Therapist is using a trigger switch to facilitate patient's dorsiflexion.

Compensatory Movement Patterns

With decreases in strength, any techniques that facilitate movement using less effort will take on greater importance. As already indicated, the SCI patient not only has decreases in strength but is usually confronted with many other physical deficits that increase the difficulty of movement; therefore, it is not surprising that compensatory movement patterns play a major role in ADL training. Maximum independence often depends on the patient's use of these patterns.

Any treatment planning process should include an understanding of what alternative movement patterns are available and how these can be applied to specific patients. This will enable the therapist and patient to decide on possible movement options early and enable the therapist to plan a program that will include development of the needed patterns.

The underlying principles for many of these movement patterns can be found in an understanding of basic anatomy and mechanics. What is the structure of our skeletal system? What motions are available at each joint, under both normal and pathological conditions? What part do ligaments and tendons play at the joint? What are the shapes and locations of all the various muscles of the body? How do their functions relate to each other? Where is the center of gravity in the body? What are gravity, friction, and inertia and how can they be related to the SCI patient?

Only a few of the many examples as to how answers to questions such as these can be specifically applied to this patient population will be discussed.

ANATOMY

Elbow Locking

The structure of the elbow joint does not allow the elbow to extend past neutral. Because of this, a quadriplegic patient may be able to bear weight on extended elbows in sitting even though he has no triceps function. With extension and external rotation at the shoulders, the elbow joint is placed in a position in which it can rely on the structure of the joint itself rather than on the triceps to provide stability.

This understanding of the elbow joint can be incorporated into many other areas of treatment programs. It may, for instance, be used to facilitate rolling. The SCI patient often uses exaggerated motions of the upper trunk and arms to move the rest of his body. Limited strength frequently requires him to rely on momentum to create some of these motions. If his arms can be maintained in extension, he effectively has a longer lever arm and is able more easily to build momentum and thus roll. Because of the elbow joint construction, upper extremity extension can be maintained even without triceps. If the patient is lying on his back, gravity is always pulling his arms down; and if his shoulders are externally rotated, this pull of gravity can be used to maintain elbow extension with up to 30 to 40 degrees of shoulder flexion. Elbow joint construction does not permit extreme hypertension.

Head/Hips Relationship

Because all the trunk is connected, movement of the head and upper trunk will have an effect on the pelvis and the lower trunk. An inverse relationship exists.

The person in Figure 4–1 is able to achieve a higher lift if he accentuates head and upper trunk flexion. Looking down and away will bring his hip up and in the W/C with greater ease. (*Note:* The movement will also provide a quick stretch to the back extensors and latissimus dorsi, which will also facilitate a higher lift.)

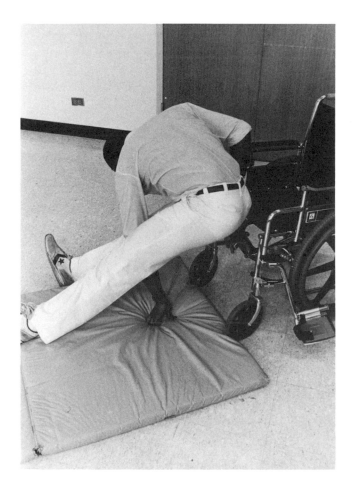

Figure 4–1 This patient uses exaggerated head flexion and the vertical positioning of his arms to achieve a higher lift.

APPLIED MECHANICS

Inertia (Newton's First Law)

It is easier to keep an object moving than to start it moving. W/C propulsion will have more speed if the patient is able to initiate the next push before the wheel has completely stopped moving. Less energy is required in a sliding board transfer if the patient is able to use two or three long pushes rather than nine or ten short pushes.

Momentum (Newton's Second Law)

One way in which to compensate for decreases in strength is to use momentum. Less effort may be required if the speed of the movement is increased. For instance, the SCI patient often does not have enough strength to lift his lower extremity onto the bed after a transfer. In one method of doing this, the patient fixes a loop around his legs and then hooks it into his bent elbow. He falls backward onto the bed, pulling his legs with him. The momentum created from his body weight being thrown quickly backward in conjunction with the force of gravity is the force used to lift his legs, not the strength of his arms.

Friction (Newton's Third Law)

Increased friction makes movement more difficult. This becomes a particularly important consideration when teaching transfers. Some types of clothing create more friction than others. Cushions vary in the amount of friction they create. The type of sliding board and the placement of that board can also be important at this point. A telescoping sliding board, for instance, has to be positioned in such a way that very little board is under the patient. The patient has to begin his slide on the cushion, which usually creates more friction than a board; therefore, even though the placement of the sliding board may be easier, the actual slide of the transfer may be more difficult.

Vectors

Consider the horizontal and vertical components of the force being used to move an object. The patient in Figure 4–1 needs a high lift to move from the floor to the W/C. Notice his arm placement. The arm on the W/C has the elbow pointing straight up and the arm on the floor is moved in between the legs. This ensures that most of the force is in a vertical direction. The horizontal components are minimized, and a higher lift is achieved.

If, on the other hand, the patient does not have enough strength to produce a strong vertical line of force and accomplish a lift, he may instead need to angle his force line more (Figure 4–2). This will incorporate more horizontal force components and make a slide easier to accomplish.

Levers

A machine is a device used to make work easier. Frequently the mechanical principles of simple machines can be applied to the body to make the work of movement easier. One simple machine that can easily be applied to the body is a lever.

All levers involve a fulcrum or a fixed point around which movement occurs, a weight to lift, and a force to lift the weight. Levers are further defined according to the placement of these three components in relation to each other.

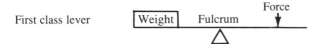

First class lever

The first class lever has the fulcrum between the weight and the force. This concept can be used to move the buttocks backward in the W/C seat. The knees act as the fulcrum. The buttocks are the weight. Bringing the head and upper trunk forward will act as part of the force that is needed to move the weight. A small additional force is needed, but the buttocks can now be easily moved back either by the patient, who can hook his thumbs into the front armrest struts and push back, or by an assistant, who simply needs to provide a small lift back at the hips.

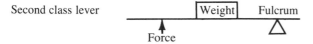

Second class lever

The second class lever has the weight between the fulcrum and the force. This mechanical principle can be used with a quadriplegic patient to assist him into sitting (Figure 4–3).

In this case, the fulcrum is at the patient's hips; the weight is in his upper trunk and the force is the pull of the biceps and upper extremity muscles.

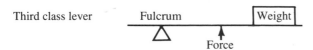

Third class lever

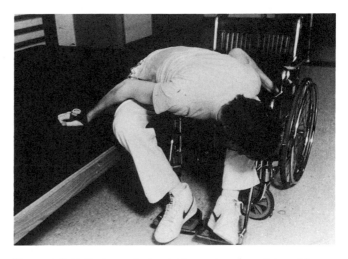

Figure 4–2 Patient uses horizontal forces to accomplish a slide.

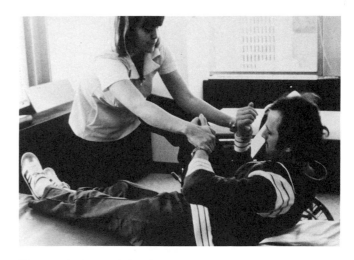

Figure 4–3 A second class lever is being used to assist the patient to a sitting position.

The patient in Figure 4–4 is using a third class lever. This time the fulcrum is at the shoulder. The force of the upper extremity is lifting the weight of the leg. *Note:* The weight is always lifted with greater difficulty if either the distance between the weight and the fulcrum is lengthened or the distance between the force and the fulcrum is shortened. This is why it is easier for the patient in Figure 4–5 to move his left leg with his right elbow resting on the right knee. This moves the fulcrum from the shoulder to the elbow, making the distance between the fulcrum and the weight (leg) shorter.

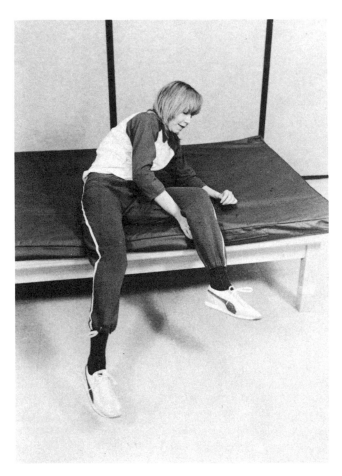

Figure 4–4 Patient uses a third class lever to lift her leg onto the mat.

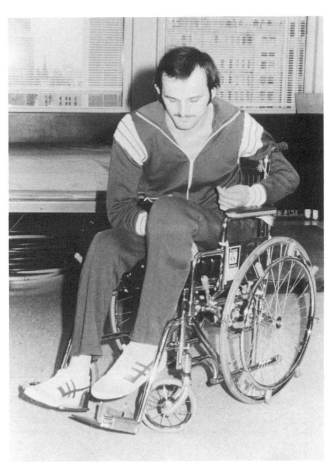

Figure 4–5 Patient uses a third class lever to lift his leg. Note the short distance between the fulcrum (elbow) and the weight (leg).

Respiration

Breathing is basically a matter of changing pressure gradients. Inspiration occurs when intrathoracic pressure is less than extrathoracic pressure. Decreased intrathoracic pressure is accomplished through muscles that act to enlarge the thoracic cavity.

During inspiration the diaphragm contracts and descends into the abdomen, enlarging the thoracic cavity both vertically and transversely. The external intercostals assist the diaphragm by increasing the anterior-posterior diameter of the upper thoracic cavity and the transverse diameter of the lower thoracic cavity. The accessory muscles tend to elevate the ribs and increase the anterior-posterior diameter. These muscles usually assist respiration through reverse action once their proximal insertions have been stabilized.

Expiration is initiated by the passive elastic recoil of the abdominal wall, which has been stretched as the diaphragm pushes down into the abdominal cavity. This decreases intrathoracic volume and increases intrathoracic pressure, forcing the air out of the chest cavity.

If the cord is transected above the C3 level, the patient has lost innervation of the phrenic nerve and thus the ability to initiate inspiration. Survival is accomplished only through an artificial life support system (e.g., artificial ventilation, phrenic stimulator) and/or the use of GPB and upper accessory muscles, when present.

If the cord is transected below the C3 level, the patient has the ability to inspire through the action of the diaphragm and accessory muscles; however, depending on the levels of injury, he probably lacks abdominal muscle tone and therefore expiration is impaired, especially forced expiration. In addition, decreased abdominal muscle tone allows the intestines to bulge through the abdominal wall, permitting the diaphragm to assume a lower position in the chest. Contractions of the diaphragm produce less excursion, particularly in the lateral chest wall, and thus inspiratory capacity is also decreased.

As is always the case, functional goals need to be established before a comprehensive respiratory program can be developed. Two primary goals exist: (1) adequate bronchial hygiene and (2) adequate coordination of good breathing skills with functional activities (Figure 5–1). Without an adequate VC neither of these goals will be achieved. Adequate VC requires good ROM and strength of the trunk musculature and the respiratory apparatus. What treatment programs can be developed to meet these goals?

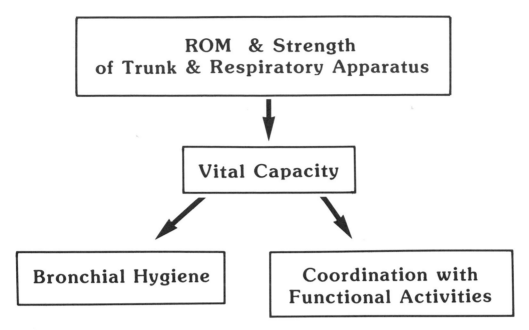

Figure 5–1 Treatment Approach

ACHIEVING THE GOAL: RESPIRATORY TREATMENT TECHNIQUES*

Improved Chest Mobility

As noted earlier, ROM deficits are often present. Treatment programs frequently begin here. Unless a joint has some range in which to move, increases in strength will have little functional meaning.

Improved ROM can be accomplished in a variety of ways. Passive manual stretches and joint mobilization techniques can be applied to the chest wall. Airshifts can also be taught. (This is a maneuver in which the patient inhales maximally and then shifts his air to various segments of the thorax.)

It is important to remember, however, that new activities do not necessarily have to be created to achieve this goal. The goal can frequently be met in already existing mat programs. For example, rolling is an activity that is included in most mat programs. The rotation used in this activity to achieve the roll will also stretch the chest wall. All static-dynamic activities involve varying amounts of weight shift and rotation. These are, perhaps, some of the best ways to mobilize

and stretch the chest, because they incorporate chest self-ROM into an already existing daily routine.

Improved Strength

Because objective testing of respiratory muscle strength is difficult, the starting points for this aspect of treatment may be less obvious. The key to this is found in looking at planes of respiratory motion. What planes of motion are being used by the patient? Does he have only inferior excursion, or is he using some anterior excursion as well? What planes of motion are limited?

Many assume that the supine posture is the best position in which to start treatment activities. Yet, in this position, anterior expansion, which is frequently difficult for patients because of intercostal deficits, is in a gravity-resisted position. If the intent of the activity is to facilitate intercostal strengthening and improve anterior excursion, it might be more appropriate to begin in a sidelying position. In this posture, anterior excursion is in a gravity-eliminated position.

Respiratory programs should be no different than other exercise programs. Activities should still progress from the easiest to the hardest. As muscles gain more strength they should be given activities that act against gravity and then progressed to activities that will provide more resistance.

Inspirometers are only one example of an activity that will provide more resistance. Any number of dif-

---

*The techniques described in this section were developed primarily by Mary Massery, P.T., and are expanded on in a chapter (in print) in the next edition of Frownfelter, D.L., *Chest Physical Therapy and Pulmonary Rehabilitation*, Chicago: Yearbook Medical Publishers, Inc., 1978.

ferent games can also be used: Who can hold their breath the longest? Who can sip punch through the most straws? Who can whistle the loudest? Who can whistle the longest? Who can count the highest in one breath? Who can blow the ping-pong ball off the table?

Improved VC

In addition to increasing ROM and strength, other things can be done to improve VC. Abdominal binders can be used to assume some of the function of the weak or absent abdominals. These can help hold the contents of the abdominal cavity up against the diaphragm, pushing the diaphragm up to a higher resting position within the chest cavity, which will in turn allow for maximal inferior and lateral excursion and increase VC.

Because of poor respiratory reserve, poor posture will have a greater impact on respiration (Figure 5–2). Correcting a kyphotic posture will help open up the chest and increase VC (Figure 5–3). Careful attention to maintaining the normal vertebral curves will help place the ribs in their optimal position for movement and again increase VC.

Trunk stabilization is another important consideration at this point. Before the accessory muscles can be used to assist in respiration, the trunk must be stable. Therefore trunk supports might be used to provide the needed stability that will enable the chest wall to move.

Improving poor breathing patterns will also impact on VC. Decreasing a fast respiratory rate will give the patient more time to inspire and thus increase VC. Trunk counterrotation can be used effectively to achieve this goal. It is begun by passively rotating the patient's trunk with each breath. As the rate of rotation is gradually slowed, the patient's respiratory rate will often slow to match the rotation movements. (*Note:* In addition to a slowed respiratory rate, the activity can also provide a good stretch to the trunk and chest wall.)

Good breathing patterns will incorporate a balanced use of all available muscles and planes of motion. If a patient is using only his diaphragm to breathe, techniques to inhibit the diaphragm and facilitate the use of accessory muscles might be used to improve VC.

Gradually increasing the pressure into the abdomen with an inward and upward motion will force the patient to use more accessory muscles. He may, however, be very frightened initially, feeling that he cannot breathe. Increasing the pressure should be done during expiration and over a series of five to six breaths. The pressure is maintained during inspiration. More anterior and superior excursion of the chest wall should be seen as the accessory muscles begin to work.

Finally, GPB can be used to improve VC.

GPB

For the patient with poor respiratory reserve, GPB is a must. The technique can also help patients relying on artificial life support systems to alleviate some of their anxiety over mechanical malfunctions. A patient skilled in this technique is often able to shut off his

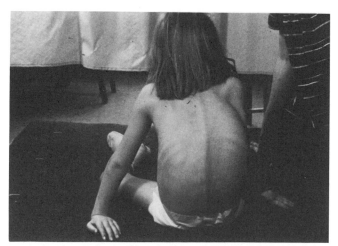

Figure 5–2 Note poor postural stabilization. The ribs will be unable to move because of poor positioning, and the accessory muscles will have trouble working effectively because of poor fixation.

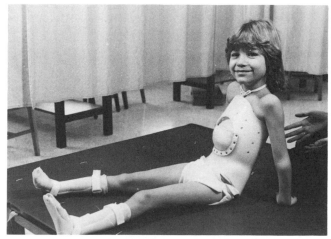

Figure 5–3 Body jacket is used to provide improved postural stabilization. An abdominal binder was not enough. Body jacket will also help minimize the scoliosis changes that are frequently seen.

support system for short periods of time and breathe on his own using GPB.

The technique is accomplished by creating the negative pressure in the buccal cavities, rather than the chest as is ordinarily done with intact musculature. As this space enlarges and negative pressure is created, air will rush in. After this occurs and the mouth is closed, the air is manually forced back and down the throat using a stroking maneuver with the tongue, pharynx, and larynx.

Teaching Procedure

After the patient understands the various uses of GPB and his specific needs for it, teaching can begin. The first step is usually just teaching the patient to hold his breath. Check to see that all nasal passages are closing.

The cervical alignment should also be checked. Small adjustments in posture can have a marked impact on success. Instruction will usually start while the patient is supine. If the patient is too weak to maintain good head and neck alignment in this position, consider providing some external support, such as a neck roll.

In any GPB instruction, it is important to keep instructions simple. Mention only those things that are necessary. This will facilitate greater continuity of movement, making the process that much easier to learn. The sound and the movements of the mouth and throat are the most important points to emphasize. Often, GPB is learned without further explanation.

The procedure can be demonstrated in the following way:

1. Take a large breath and hold it. (This eliminates the possibility of using other accessory muscles while learning the technique.)
2. Shape your lips as if to say, "oop."
3. Bring your jaw down and then forward and up as if reaching with your lips for a cherry that is held just above the upper lip.
4. Close your mouth, reaching the bottom lip to the upper lip.
5. Draw the tongue and jaw back toward the throat. (Mouth and tongue should be formed as if saying the word "up" or the sound "l." Some patients learn the maneuver by actually saying "up" as they retract the tongue.)
6. Repeat this stroke four or five times.
7. Exhale and relax.

After demonstrating for the patient, direct him to imitate the procedure. During initial attempts, it may be more comfortable for the patient to perform simultaneously with the therapist to help prevent his becoming self-conscious and keep the correct pattern in mind.

Remember that the feedback mechanisms available to a patient using this musculature are not the same as those on which he ordinarily relies for trunk and extremity muscle movements. He can't see his tongue and can't feel the isolated movements of his throat. Muscle control of many of these muscle groups is usually unconscious. So any additional feedback the therapist can provide, such as using a mirror or cuing the patient in to sounds to imitate, will greatly facilitate learning. (A spirometer can be used to measure vital capacity both with and without GPB to objectively evaluate success.)

It is best to limit the number of stroke repetitions to three or four at first. Many patients tire easily and then are unable to hold their breath. This will result in air escaping through the nose. A regular time for daily practice should be scheduled.

Potential Problems

Open Nose. Difficulty with air escaping through the nose is usually found in patients who have some ability to breath on their own rather than among those who cannot do this, indicating that the problem may be due to carelessness in holding the breath. Special attention should be given to this problem during initial training. Preventing air leaking through the nose is easier than correcting the habit once it has been established.

Incoordinate Movements. Only those movements essential to GPB should be encouraged. Some patients develop extra movements in the abdominal region or try to use head bobbing. Once these habits develop, they are difficult to break. If these movements are seen during initial training sessions, reduce the number of strokes per series to one. When the patient can easily perform one stroke without incoordinate movements, gradually increase the number of strokes in the series.

Incorrect Sounds. If the tongue is properly retracted, the sound will not be a clear "up." The tongue movement often causes an "l" sound. This is permissible. However, do not let the patient try to say "ulp" or "gulp," since the "g" and the "p" sounds destroy the rhythm. The sound of "m" is associated with loss of air through the mouth, while a "smacking" sound is associated with loss of air through the nose. The "drum" sound indicates that there is too much tension in the throat. The stroke sounds should not run together but rather should be chopped off in a staccato manner.

Building Up Endurance. As the patient begins to build up GPB endurance, flushing of the face, sweating, and/or an increased pulse rate may be noticed. This normally occurs any time endurance is upgraded with new activities. Avoid calling the patient's attention to these features.

Building up GPB endurance should be done gradually and in a systematic way. Do not let the patient do 5 minutes of GPB one day and 20 minutes the next. GPB should not be attempted in a sitting position until the patient is expert in the supine position. This will mean that he should be able to do an adequate cough.

Note: The techniques described above are used to facilitate the learning process. Once the patient has mastered GPB, the sound and facial movements are eliminated. Experts are able to perform silently and with only a slight movement under the chin.

ASSISTIVE COUGH TECHNIQUES

There are times when increasing ROM, strength, and VC are not enough. More specific techniques have to be learned to achieve the functional goals. Assistive coughing techniques are one example of this.

One of the most familiar assistive cough techniques is to apply firm pressure into the abdomen with an inward and upward motion while forcefully exhaling. A patient with upper extremity strength can do this himself in sitting. If upper extremity strength is limited, he may have someone assist him. This can be done in a supine, sidelying, or sitting position (Figure 5–4).

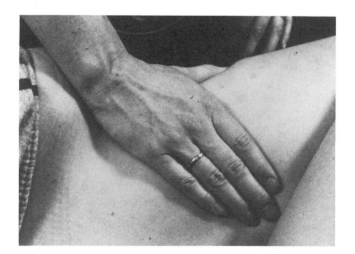

Figure 5–4 Assisted cough technique. Any quick compressive force against the chest wall will assist a cough. Compression of the lower costal ribs can be done in both sidelying and sitting positions.

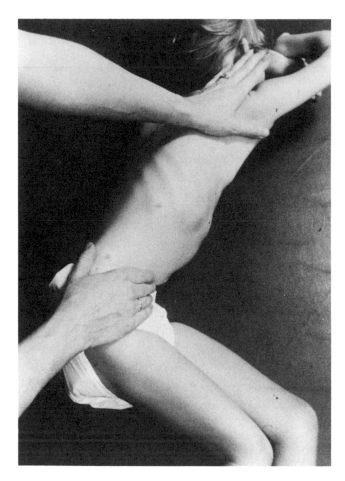

Figure 5–5a Trunk counterrotation can be used in a sidelying position to assist a cough. Note how the motion opens up the chest and how all planes of motion are stretched, facilitating increased VC.

Almost any quick movement into trunk flexion during forced exhalation will facilitate coughing (Figures 5–6a through 5–6c). Some quadriplegic patients take advantage of this principle when coughing by assuming a supine-on-elbows position, extending their head and back as they inhale and then quickly flexing forward as they exhale. This same principle can be applied to a sitting posture, both with and without upper extremity support, to assist coughing.

As with many other skills, there is no one correct method of assistive coughing. Only a few techniques have been discussed. Each patient chooses and modifies the various techniques to meet his particular situation.

Coughing can also be assisted from a sidelying position using counterrotation (Figure 5–5a). The patient inhales as the shoulders are forward and the pelvis is pulled back. As the patient exhales, the pelvis is quickly pushed forward and up and the shoulders pulled back and down (Figure 5–5b). This is often more comfortable than the pressure of a hand in the abdomen but always requires the assistance of another.

Doing a sequence of slow rotation prior to asking the patient to cough will slow the respiratory rate, relax any tone that is present, and stretch the chest wall, all of which will facilitate an increased VC and produce a more functional cough.

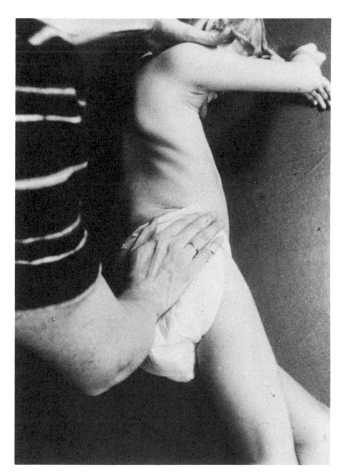

Figure 5–5b As the pelvis is quickly pushed up and forward, air is forced out of the lungs.

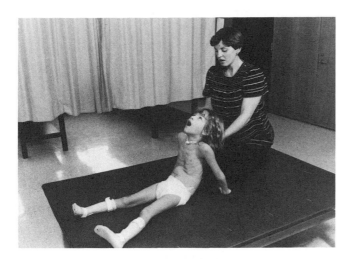

Figure 5–6a Assisted coughing is used with trunk flexion.

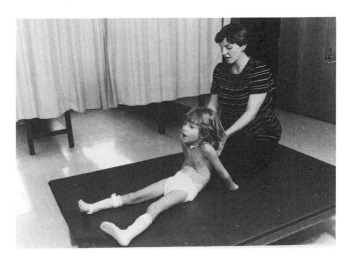

Figure 5–6b

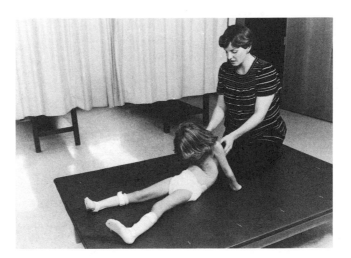

Figure 5–6c

FINAL COMMENT

Before leaving the respiratory treatment program, look back at the initially set goals. Have they been achieved? Are there other things that can be done to facilitate achievement of these ends?

In order for a patient to be able to coordinate his breathing with functional activities he must be challenged. Has this been done? If he is only taught to breathe with correct patterns while he is lying quietly, he will never be able to coordinate breathing with movement and his endurance will remain low. If phonation is still poor, consider using some vibration during expiration. This can increase the number of syllables the patient is able to say in one breath.

Is the patient able to maintain adequate bronchial hygiene? In addition to assistive coughing techniques movement is needed to mobilize secretions. Is the patient comfortable with this, or is he hesitant to move on his own or afraid of being passively moved? If suctioning is needed, can the patient direct this? Postural drainage positions and techniques should be routinely taught to those patients with a weak or nonfunctional cough.

Achievement of respiratory goals should be an integral part of any treatment program. A creative therapist will weave these into the patient care plan with skill and ease. An example of an evaluation form is presented in Appendix F, Exhibit F–3.

Respiration—C4 Quadriplegic

Outcome

1. Patient demonstrates ability to achieve a vital capacity (VC) of at least 30% to 50% of his expected norm.

2. Patient demonstrates ability to say four to six syllables per breath.

3. Patient demonstrates ability to direct his bronchial hygiene.

4. Patient demonstrates ability to coordinate respiration to achieve all other noted outcomes.

Components

a. Bronchial hygiene:
   - mobilizing secretions
   - clearing secretions from lungs

b. Coordination of respiration with functional activities:
   - operating sip and puff controls
   - directing all ADL (bed mobility, pressure relief, transfers, W/C mobility)

Considerations

1. Previous and current respiratory status:
   - allergies, asthma
   - respiratory complications related to injury
   - tracheostomy

2. Presence of pressure sores, abnormal tone, decreased ROM, and/or patient's general fear or discomfort with movement may make positioning and handling more difficult and may therefore limit techniques for bronchial hygiene.

3. Equipment: What is available to assist?
   - Abdominal binders may increase VC and assist with cough
   - Motorized reclining W/C may be considered to assist with position changes in sitting that may decrease the potential for secretion pooling

4. GPB may add as much as 1000 cc to patient's VC.

Process

1. Evaluate present respiratory status and skills (see section on respiratory evaluation).

2. Improve ROM and strength of trunk and respiratory apparatus:
   - Emphasize increased proximal joint ROM.
   - Improve chest expansion via airshifts, rotational exercises, and so on.
   - Improve strength of diaphragm and accessory muscles.

3. Improve VC by:
   - positioning
   - creating good trunk stability (consider trunk supports)
   - improved breathing patterns
   - use of abdominal binders
   - teaching GPB
   - using pool, respiratory classes, and individual sessions

4. Teach skills to improve and/or maintain good bronchial hygiene:
   - Increase patient's comfort with being handled and moved into as many different developmental postures as possible.
   - Teach assisted coughing techniques.
   - Teach suctioning techniques.
   - Consider teaching postural drainage.

5. Coordinate respiration with functional activities.

6. Instruct nursing staff, other team members, and significant others in respiratory skills.

7. Incorporate skills into daily routine.

8. Evaluate performance in daily routine.

9. Assist patient in problem solving to alleviate difficulties.

Respiration—C5 Quadriplegic

Outcome

1. Patient demonstrates ability to achieve a VC of at least *40 to 60%* of his expected norm.

2. Patient demonstrates ability to say six to eight *syllables per breath*.

3. Patient demonstrates ability to direct/*assist* with bronchial hygiene.

4. Patient demonstrates ability to coordinate respiration to achieve all other noted outcomes (at his level).

Components

a. Bronchial hygiene:

   - mobilizing secretions
   - clearing secretions from lungs

b. Coordination of respiration and functional activities:

   - operating sip and puff controls and/or *hand control*
   - *assisting*/directing all ADL (bed mobility, pressure relief, transfers, W/C mobility)

Considerations

1. Previous and current respiratory status:

   - allergies, asthma
   - respiratory complications related to injury
   - tracheostomy

2. Presence of pressure sores, abnormal tone, decreased ROM, and/or patient's general fear or discomfort with movement may make positioning and handling more difficult and may therefore limit techniques for bronchial hygiene.

3. Equipment: What is available to assist?

   - Abdominal binders may increase VC and assist with cough.
   - Motorized reclining W/C may be considered to assist with position changes in sitting that may decrease the potential for secretion pooling.

4. GPB may add as much as 1000 cc to patient's VC.

Process

1. Evaluate present respiratory status and skills (see section on respiratory evaluation).

2. Improve ROM and strength of trunk and respiratory apparatus:

   - Emphasize increased proximal joint ROM.
   - Improve chest expansion via airshifts, rotational exercises, and so on.
   - Improve strength of diaphragm and accessory muscles.

3. Improve VC by:

   - positioning
   - creating good trunk stability (consider trunk supports)
   - improving breathing patterns
   - using abdominal binders
   - teaching GPB
   - using pool, respiratory classes, and individual sessions

4. Teach skills to improve and/or maintain good bronchial hygiene:

   - Increase patient's comfort with being handled and moved into as many different developmental postures as possible.
   - Teach assisted coughing techniques.
   - Teach suctioning techniques.
   - Consider teaching postural drainage.

5. Coordinate respiration with functional activities.

6. Instruct nursing staff, other team members, and significant others in respiratory skills.

7. Incorporate skills into daily routine.

8. Evaluate performance in daily routine.

9. Assist patient in problem solving to alleviate difficulties.

Respiration—C6 Quadriplegic

Outcome

1. Patient demonstrates ability to achieve a VC of at least *60% to 80%* of his expected norm.

2. Patient demonstrates ability to say *eight syllables per breath*.

3. Patient demonstrates ability to *assist/perform* bronchial hygiene.

4. Patient demonstrates ability to coordinate respiration to achieve all other noted outcomes.

Components

a. Bronchial hygiene:

   - mobilizing secretions
   - clearing secretions from lungs

b. Coordination of respiration with functional activities:

   - assisting/*performing* all ADL from W/C level (bed mobility, pressure relief, transfers, W/C mobility [with the exception of advanced W/C skills])

Considerations

1. Previous and current respiratory status:

   - allergies, asthma
   - respiratory complications related to injury
   - tracheostomy

2. Presence of pressure sores, abnormal tone, decreased ROM, and/or patient's general discomfort with movement may make positioning more difficult and may therefore limit techniques for bronchial hygiene.

3. Equipment: What is available to assist?

   - Abdominal binders may increase VC and assist with cough.

4. GPB may add as much as 1000 cc to patient's VC.

5. *Age*

Process

1. Evaluate present respiratory status and skills (see section on respiratory evaluation).

2. Improve ROM and strength of trunk and respiratory apparatus:

   - Emphasize increased proximal joint ROM.
   - Improve chest expansion via airshifts, rotational exercises, and so on.
   - Improve strength of diaphragm and accessory muscles as appropriate.

3. Improve VC by:

   - positioning
   - creating good trunk stability
   - improving breathing patterns
   - using abdominal binders
   - teaching GPB
   - using pool, respiratory classes, and individual sessions

4. Teach skills to improve and/or maintain good bronchial hygiene:

   - Teach assisted coughing techniques.
   - *Teach movement patterns to mobilize secretions.*
   - Consider teaching postural drainage.

5. Coordinate respiration with functional activities.

6. Instruct nursing staff, other team members, and significant others in respiratory skills.

7. Incorporate skills into daily routine.

8. Evaluate performance in daily routine.

9. Assist patient in problem solving to alleviate difficulties.

Respiration—C7–8 Quadriplegic

Outcome

1. Patient demonstrates ability to achieve a VC of at least 60% to 80% of his expected norm.

2. Patient demonstrates ability to say eight syllables per breath.

3. Patient demonstrates ability to *perform* bronchial hygiene.

4. Patient demonstrates ability to coordinate respiration to achieve all other noted outcomes.

Components

a. Bronchial hygiene:

  • mobilizing secretions
  • clearing secretions from lungs

b. Coordination of respiration with functional activities:

  • *independent performance* of all ADL from W/C level (bed mobility, pressure relief, transfers, W/C mobility [with the possible exception of advanced W/C skills])

Considerations

1. Previous and current respiratory status:

  • allergies, asthma
  • respiratory complications related to injury

2. Presence of pressure sores, abnormal tone, decreased ROM, and/or patient's general discomfort with movement may make positioning and handling more difficult and may therefore limit techniques for bronchial hygiene.

3. Equipment: What is available to assist?

  • Abdominal binders may increase VC and assist with cough.

4. GPB may add as much as 1000 cc to patient's VC.

5. Age.

Process

1. Evaluate present respiratory status and skills (see section on respiratory evaluation).

2. Improve ROM and strength of trunk and respiratory apparatus:

  • Emphasize increased proximal joint ROM.
  • Improve chest expansion via airshifts, rotational exercises, and so on.
  • Improve strength of diaphragm and accessory muscles as appropriate.

3. Improve VC by:

  • positioning
  • creating good trunk stability
  • improving breathing patterns
  • using abdominal binders
  • using pool, respiratory classes, and individual sessions

4. Teach skills to improve and/or maintain good bronchial hygiene:

  • Teach assisted coughing techniques.
  • Teach movement patterns to mobilize secretions.
  • Consider teaching postural drainage.

5. Coordinate respiration with functional activities.

6. Instruct nursing staff, other team members, and significant others in respiratory skills.

7. Incorporate skills into daily routine.

8. Evaluate performance in daily routine.

9. Assist patient in problem solving to alleviate difficulties.

Respiration—Paraplegic

Outcome

1. Patient demonstrates ability to achieve a *VC of 80%* of his expected norm.

2. Patient demonstrates independent performance of bronchial hygiene.

3. Patient demonstrates ability to coordinate respiration to achieve all other noted outcomes.

Components

a. Bronchial hygiene:

   • mobilizing secretions
   • clearing secretions from lungs

b. Coordination of respiration with functional activities:

   • independent performance of all ADL (bed mobility, pressure relief, transfers, W/C mobility, *ambulation [as indicated]*)

Considerations

1. Previous and current respiratory status:

   • allergies, asthma
   • respiratory complications related to injury

2. Presence of pressure sores, abnormal tone, decreased ROM, and/or patient's general discomfort with movement may make positioning and handling more difficult and may therefore limit techniques for bronchial hygiene.

3. Age.

Process

1. Evaluate present respiratory status and skills (see section on respiratory evaluation).

2. Improve ROM and strength of trunk and respiratory apparatus:

   • Emphasize increased proximal joint ROM.
   • Improve chest expansion via airshifts, rotational exercises, and so on.
   • Improve strength of diaphragm and accessory muscles as appropriate.

3. Improve VC by:

   • improving breathing patterns
   • using abdominal binders
   • using pool, respiratory classes, and individual sessions

4. Teach skills to improve and/or maintain good bronchial hygiene:

   • Teach coughing techniques.
   • Teach movement patterns to mobilize secretions.

5. Coordinate respiration with functional activities.

6. Instruct nursing staff, other team members, and significant others in respiratory skills.

7. Incorporate skills into daily routine.

8. Evaluate performance in daily routine.

9. Assist patient in problem solving to alleviate difficulties.

Bed Mobility

As with most ADL, many possible ways of accomplishing each aspect of bed mobility exist. The method used will depend on the patient's "body English," his discharge plans, and his particular needs. The following are examples of possible ways to approach the various aspects of bed mobility.

ACHIEVING THE OUTCOME

Rolling

A patient often begins to learn rolling in a sidelying position using scapula and upper trunk movement. The therapist can facilitate learning by assisting and/or resisting the forward and backward motion of the shoulders.

The next step is to combine shoulder flexion with scapula abduction and scapula adduction with shoulder extension. The increased movement of the shoulders and upper trunk plus the leverage provided by the extended upper extremities add to the momentum generated.

Cuff weights placed at the wrist will reinforce the correct movement patterns and facilitate rolling. The therapist may vary the amount of weight according to individual patient needs. Increasing the weight will provide greater *resistance* to muscle groups but greater *assistance* to the rolling activity. Reducing the weight will have the opposite effect: less *resistance* to muscle groups and less *assistance* to rolling. These activities help to make the patient more aware of how lower trunk motion can be achieved by exaggerated movement of the upper extremities and trunk.

The patient can practice rolling independently, without the aid of cuff weights. A pillow placed behind his hips to limit posterior motion of the pelvis will make rolling easier initially. As more skill is gained, he will eventually be able to initiate the movement without the pillow.

Leg position also affects the degree of difficulty in rolling. Rolling is easiest with one or both knees flexed. As the patient progresses, the knees can be extended with the legs crossed. Rolling is most difficult to accomplish with the legs both extended and uncrossed.

If the patient is unable to generate enough momentum to effect a roll, he may still be able to accomplish the task by pulling on the bed side rails.

Movement on the Bed in a Supine Position

The patient who is unable to move on the bed using only his head and the remaining muscle power of his arms and/or legs can often accomplish the task by pulling on the side rails. Loops placed at various places on the rail may facilitate the movement.

The patient may also want to consider planning more carefully to which part of the bed he wishes to transfer. This will avoid unnecessary movement up and down the bed once on it. If the patient transfers to the bed near the foot of the bed, he will then be able to straighten out his legs with the same movement he uses to pull up to the head of the bed.

Assuming Prone-on-Elbows Posture

Mobility within a prone-on-elbows posture can be used to assist in bed positioning and to assume a sitting position.

To assume the position, the patient may begin with his hands near his shoulders and his elbows close to his trunk. He then pushes his elbows onto the mat, lifting the upper trunk. The final position is achieved in one of two ways: either the patient shifts his weight from side to side moving his elbows up under his shoulders (Figures 6–1a through 6–1e) or he pushes his entire body backward until his elbows are under the shoulders (Figures 6–2a and 6–2b).

Some patients seem to find it easier to start with one arm extended over the head and the other flexed with the hand at the shoulder and elbow into the side. As above, the patient then pushes into the mat, lifts the upper trunk, and shifts his weight from side to side as he moves his elbows under the shoulders.

Supine-on-Elbows Posture

Like the prone-on-elbows posture, the supine-on-elbows posture can be used to assist in bed positioning and to assume a sitting position. However, this position is often more difficult to assume than the prone-on-elbows position.

Some patients are able simply to dig their elbows into the mat and "muscle up" into this position. However, this method is often impossible for the patient without abdominal muscles. Such a patient may be able to assume the position by first rolling to one side and coming up on his bottom elbow. As he rolls back to the supine position, he quickly extends his top arm and places the elbow under the shoulder. He then shifts his weight onto this extremity and positions the other elbow under his shoulder. This requires good speed and timing (Figures 6–3a through 6–3e).

Many patients are able to assume supine-on-elbows posture by placing their hands under their hips or hooking their thumbs into their pockets. By using their wrist extensors and/or their biceps, they are able to pull halfway up into the posture. Then, as they shift their weight from side to side, they are able to reposition their elbows under the shoulders (Figures 6–4a through 6–4d).

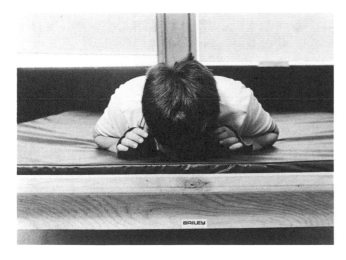

Figure 6–1a Patient assumes a prone-on-elbow posture.

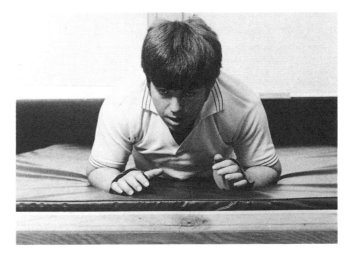

Figure 6–1b

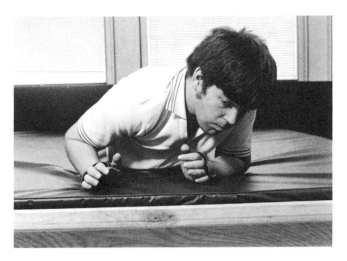

Figure 6–1c

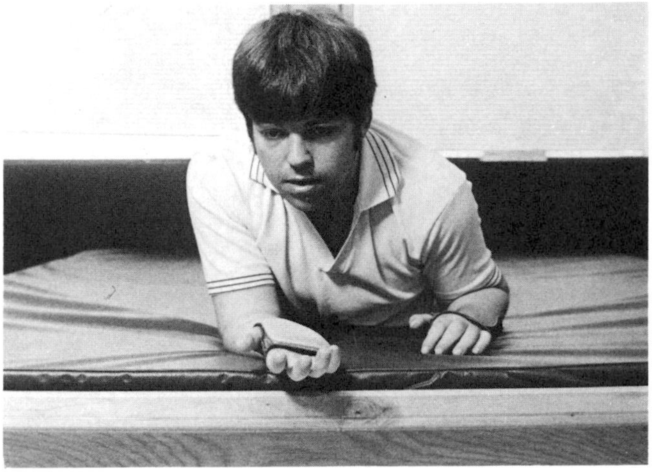

Figure 6–1d

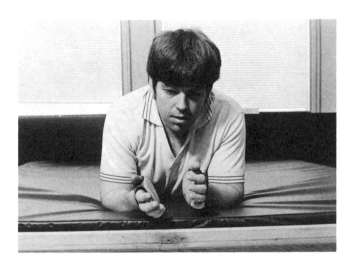

Figure 6–1e

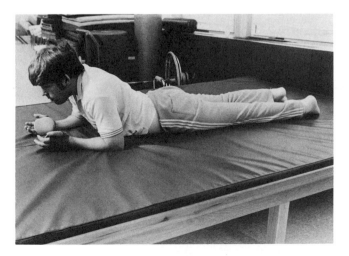

Figure 6–2a Patient assumes a prone-on-elbows posture. Patient achieves the final position by pushing his body backward until the elbows are under the shoulders.

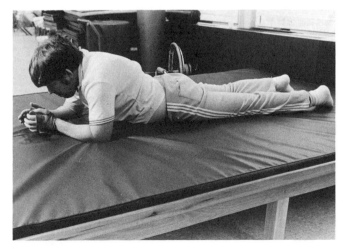

Figure 6–2b

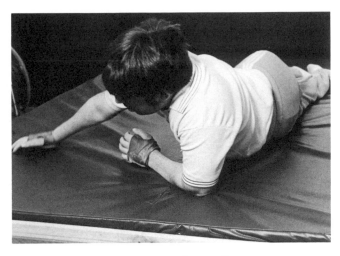

Figure 6–3a Patient assumes a supine-on-elbows posture.

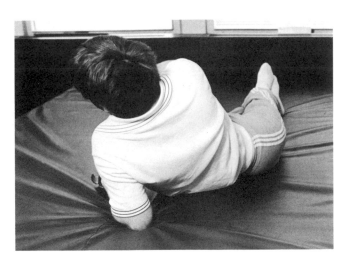

Figure 6–3b

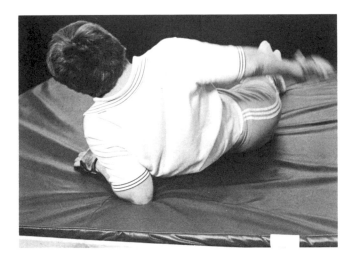

Figure 6–3c

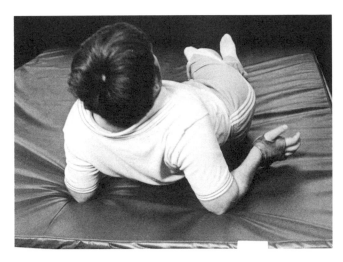

Figure 6–3d

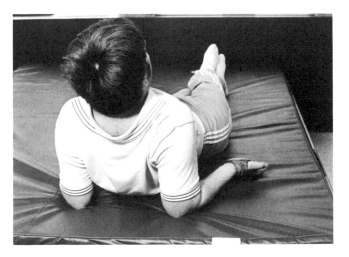

Figure 6–3e

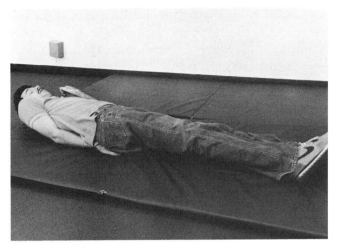

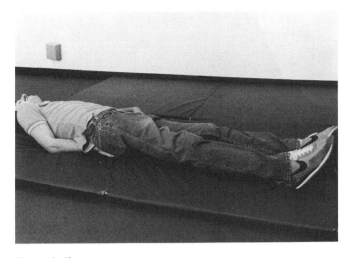

Figure 6–4a Patient assumes supine-on-elbows posture using his biceps to pull against his hips.

Figure 6–4b

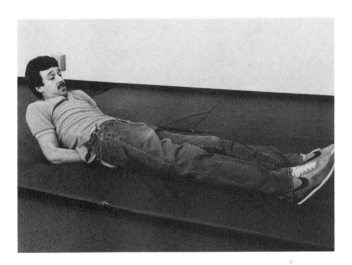

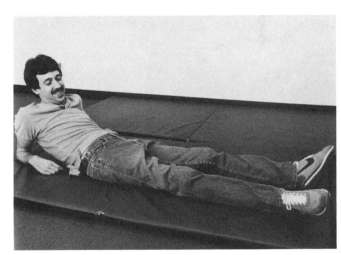

Figure 6–4c

Figure 6–4d

Figures 6–5a through 6–5d show yet another way to achieve the supine-on-elbows position. This patient uses the momentum of forcefully flexing his arms and head to curl forward and then he quickly throws his elbows back to position them under his shoulders.

Sitting

With abdominals and triceps, most patients are able to push on their arms directly into sitting from the su-pine position. Without abdominal muscles, a patient may first roll into sidelying placing his lower arm under his head and the upper arm on the mat. From here, he is able to push with his triceps up to sitting.

If the triceps muscle group is not intact, the patient is usually forced to start in one of two positions: supine-on-elbows or prone-on-elbows.

From a supine-on-elbows position, the patient be-gins by rocking from side to side, attempting to build up

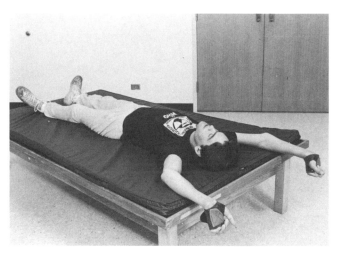

Figure 6–5a Assuming supine on elbows.

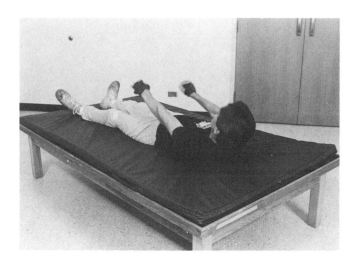

Figure 6–5b

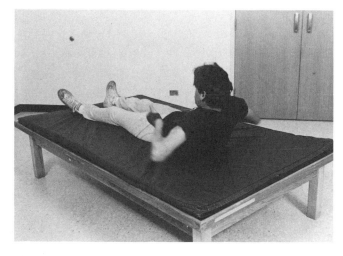

Figure 6–5c

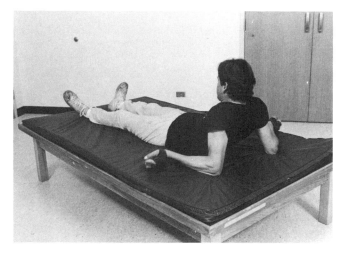

Figure 6–5d

enough momentum to throw one arm behind and immediately shift his weight onto this extended arm. He is then able to throw the other arm behind him and walk up on extended arms to a sitting position. The momentum of "throwing" the arms back helps extend the elbows; this position can then be maintained by the pectoralis muscles with the shoulder placed in extension and external rotation (Figures 6–6a through 6–6d).

If the patient uses the prone-on-elbows posture as his starting position, he "walks" around to the side using his forearms and head, if necessary. When he is curled into a C curve, he uses one arm to hook under his knee. As he pulls with this arm, he flings the other arm behind him, locking the elbow into extension. The first arm is then thrown behind him, and the patient walks with his extended arms the rest of the way up to sitting. There are many variations on this theme. The patient in Figures 6–7a through 6–7f has more flexibility in his trunk. He, too, walks around to the side and hooks his arm around his knees, but he uses this pull to bring his remaining elbow up in front of his hips. From here he is able to push straight up to sitting.

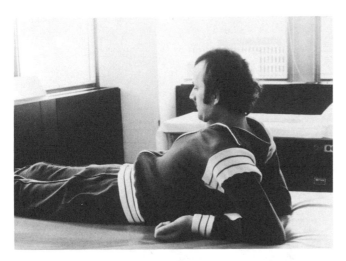

Figure 6–6a Patient assumes sitting position from a supine-on-elbows position.

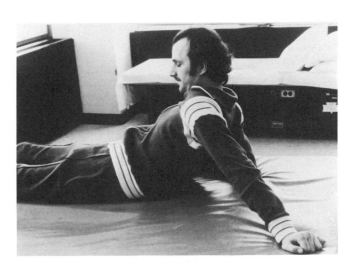

Figure 6–6b

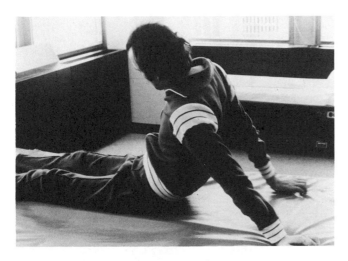

Figure 6–6c

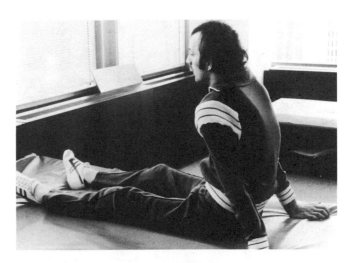

Figure 6–6d

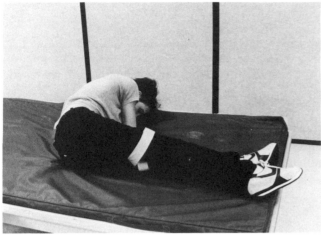

Figure 6–7a Patient assumes sitting position using a modified prone-on-elbows position.

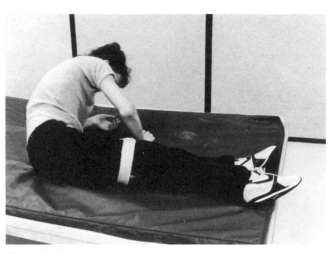

Figure 6–7b

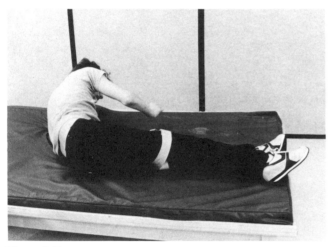

Figure 6–7c

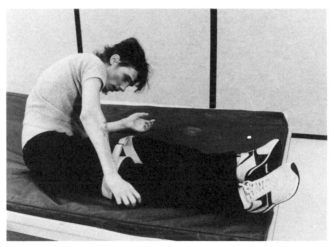

Figure 6–7d

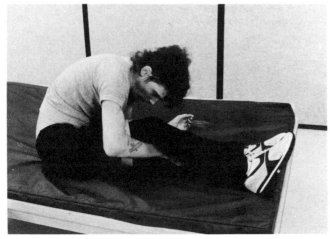

Figure 6–7e

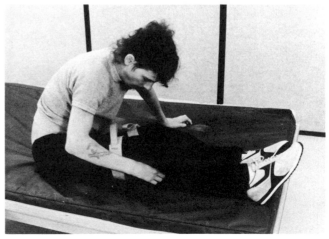

Figure 6–7f

EQUIPMENT OPTIONS

Not all individuals will need a hospital bed. However, if a patient can be more independent in transfers, bed mobility, dressing, or catheterization, use of a hospital bed can be justified. The age and health of the primary care giver should also be a consideration in this decision.

Both manual and electric hospital beds are available, and a double electric bed can also be ordered if needed. The features of two types of electric beds are compared in Table 6–1.

On both beds, the mattresses must be ordered separately. The foam mattress is usually the one preferred. Although the innerspring mattresses are firmer, they do not bend or fold well in hospital beds. Springs can break through the mattress and pose a potential hazard to insensitive skin. If a firmer mattress is preferred, some choose not to buy a hospital bed and order a commercially available mattress for a regular bed.

Occasionally, requests are made for waterbeds. Although they may aid in skin care, waterbeds tend to reduce independence in bed mobility and transfers. The Rochester mattress has been used as a compromise. This mattress provides water pockets under vulnerable skin areas but does not seem to decrease independence levels as drastically as the commercially available waterbeds.

A portable trapeze can be used on conventional beds; however, these will not swivel. If a swivel bar transfer is used, a hospital bed needs to be ordered.

Side rails can be applied to regular beds as well as hospital beds.

TABLE 6–1   Comparison of Electric Hospital Beds

	Borg-Warner	*Smith-Davis*
Durability	Both beds have comparable durability.	
Cosmesis	Many prefer this bed because it looks less like a hospital bed.	
Comfort	An 18-inch extension for the tall individual is available.	
Function	Motor seems to have more power than Smith-Davis, which may be a consideration for the obese patient or when using water mattresses.	It weighs 220 pounds, comes apart in three pieces, and is easily moved.
	It weighs 550 pounds, comes in one piece, and is difficult to move.	
ADL Mobility During transfer	Lowest position is 20 inches from floor (without casters), so independent sliding board transfers may be more difficult.	Lowest position is 19 inches from floor (without casters); transfers to and from are usually easier, and more transfer approaches are possible.
	Casters can be taken off to facilitate easier lateral transfers (but makes use of mechanical lifts impossible since legs will not fit under bed).	
	Trapeze cannot be hooked onto headboard, so swivel bar transfers are not an option.	
In bed	Side rails do not come up as the head of the bed is raised; those who rely on rails to move in bed will be less mobile.	Side rails come up as head of bed is raised.
		Hand controls have recessed area for buttons; those with limited hand function find this easier to manipulate than the Borg-Warner.

Bed Mobility—C4 Quadriplegic

Outcome

1. Patient demonstrates ability to move independently from supine to sitting and back using electric bed (patient will not be able to use upper extremities for control).

2. Patient demonstrates ability to provide occasional minimal assist using head and scapular movements with other bed mobility.

3. Patient demonstrates ability to direct all bed mobility.

Components

a. Rolling to right and left

b. Rolling from prone to supine and back

c. Moving from supine to sitting (both long sitting and short sitting) and return to supine

d. Moving to either side of the bed

e. Moving to head and foot of the bed

f. Performing pressure relief in bed

Considerations

1. Strength, especially:
   - neck musculature
   - available movement patterns

2. ROM: normal ROM particularly important at:
   - shoulders
   - hips

3. Tone

4. Respiratory status as it relates to ability to direct care

5. Existing pressure sores and/or fragile skin (may make activity more difficult)

6. Equipment: What is available to assist?
   - type of bed
   - type of controls (air switch, chin control, voice control)

7. Personality prior to injury:
   - How assertive was patient?

Process

1. Evaluate motor skills.

2. Evaluate functional component skills:
   - head control
   - comfort with being handled and moved
   - respiratory skills needed to direct care
   - manipulation of bed controls

3. Improve motor skills.

4. Improve functional component skills.

5. Determine appropriate bed mobility techniques; consult with OT and speech therapist.

6. Evaluate potential equipment needs.

7. Teach bed mobility skills.

8. Determine equipment needs.

9. Instruct nursing staff, OT, and significant others in patient's bed mobility skills.

10. Incorporate skills into daily routine.

11. Evaluate performance in daily routine.

12. Assist patient in problem solving to alleviate difficulties.

Bed Mobility—C5 Quadriplegic

Outcome

1. Patient demonstrates ability to move independently from supine to sitting and back using electric bed (*patient may be able to use some type of upper extremity control*).

2. Patient demonstrates ability to provide *moderate assist* using head, scapular movements and/or shoulder movements, with other bed mobility.

3. Patient demonstrates ability to direct all bed mobility.

Components

a. Rolling to right and left

b. Rolling from prone to supine and back

c. Moving from supine to sitting (both long sitting and short sitting) and return to supine

d. Moving to either side of the bed

e. Moving to head and foot of the bed

f. Performing pressure relief in bed

Considerations

1. Strength, especially:

   - neck musculature
   - *scapular musculature*
   - *pectoralis major*
   - *elbow flexors*

2. ROM: normal ROM particularly important at:

   - shoulders
   - hips

3. Tone

4. Respiratory status as it relates to ability to direct care

5. Existing pressure sores and/or fragile skin (may make activity more difficult)

6. Equipment: What is available to assist?

   - type of bed
   - type of controls
   - *side rails* (may find it easier to pull on some designs than others)
   - *loops and straps*
   - *mattress* (firmer ones are usually easier to move on)

7. Personality prior to injury:

   - How assertive was patient?

Process

1. Evaluate motor skills.

2. Evaluate functional component skills:

   - head control
   - comfort with being handled and moved
   - respiratory skills needed to direct care
   - manipulation of bed controls
   - *weight shift in lower development postures*
   - *balance and equilibrium reactions in sidelying and on elbows*
   - *compensatory movement patterns to compensate for absent musculature*
   - *compensatory sensory techniques*
   - *skills to compensate for abnormal tone*

3. Improve motor skills.

4. Improve functional component skills.

5. Determine appropriate bed mobility techniques.

6. Evaluate potential equipment needs.

7. Teach bed mobility skills.

8. Determine equipment needs.

9. Instruct nursing staff, OT, and significant others in patient's bed mobility skills.

10. Incorporate skills into daily routine.

11. Evaluate performance in daily routine.

12. Assist patient in problem solving to alleviate difficulties.

Bed Mobility—C6 Quadriplegic

Outcome

1. Patient demonstrates *ability to perform bed mobility independently with or without side rails.*

Components

a. Rolling to right and left

b. Rolling from prone to supine and back

c. Moving from supine to sitting (both long sitting and short sitting) and return to supine

d. Moving to either side of the bed

e. Moving to head and foot of the bed

f. Performing pressure relief in bed

Considerations

1. Strength, especially:

   - *shoulders, depressors*
   - pectoralis major
   - elbow flexors
   - *wrist extensors*

2. ROM: normal ROM particularly important at:

   - shoulders
   - *wrists*
   - hips

3. Tone

4. *Coordination: patient's ability to learn new movement patterns*

5. *Endurance: independence can require high endurance levels*

6. Existing pressure sores and/or fragile skin (may make activity more difficult and/or delay training)

7. Equipment: What is available to assist?

   - *electric bed may be considered to conserve energy*
   - side rails, loops
   - mattress (firmer ones are usually easier to move on)

8. *Age*

9. *Obesity*

Process

1. Evaluate motor skills.

2. Evaluate functional component skills:

   - weight shift in lower developmental postures
   - balance and equilibrium reactions in sidelying and on elbows
   - compensatory movement patterns to compensate for absent musculature
   - compensatory sensory techniques
   - skills to compensate for abnormal tone

3. Improve motor skills.

4. Improve functional component skills.

5. Determine appropriate bed mobility techniques.

6. Evaluate potential equipment needs.

7. Teach bed mobility skills.

8. Determine equipment needs.

9. Instruct nursing staff, OT, and significant others in patient's bed mobility skills.

10. Incorporate skills into daily routine.

11. Evaluate performance in daily routine.

12. Assist patient in problem solving to alleviate difficulties.

Bed Mobility—C7–8 Quadriplegic

Outcome

1. Patient demonstrates ability to perform bed mobility independently *without special equipment*.

Components

a. Rolling to right and left

b. Rolling from prone to supine and back

c. Moving from supine to sitting (both long sitting and short sitting) and return to supine

d. Moving to either side of the bed

e. Moving to head and foot of the bed

f. Performing pressure relief in bed

Considerations

1. Strength, especially:

   - *triceps*
   - wrist extensors

2. ROM: normal ROM particularly important at:

   - shoulders
   - wrists
   - hips

3. Tone

4. Existing pressure sores and/or fragile skin (may make activity more difficult)

5. Age

6. Obesity

Process

1. Evaluate motor skills.

2. Evaluate functional component skills:

   - weight shift in lower developmental postures
   - balance and equilibrium reactions in sidelying and on elbows
   - compensatory movement patterns to compensate for absent musculature
   - compensatory sensory techniques
   - skills to compensate for abnormal tone

3. Improve motor skills.

4. Teach functional component skills.

5. Determine appropriate bed mobility techniques.

6. Evaluate potential equipment needs.

7. Teach bed mobility skills.

8. Determine equipment needs.

9. Instruct nursing staff, OT, and significant others in patient's bed mobility skills.

10. Incorporate skills into daily routine.

11. Evaluate performance in daily routine.

12. Assist patient in problem solving to alleviate difficulties.

Bed Mobility—Paraplegic

Outcome

1. Patient demonstrates ability to perform bed mobility independently *without special equipment*.

Components

a. Rolling to right and left

b. Rolling from prone to supine and back

c. Moving from supine to sitting (both long sitting and short sitting) and return to supine

d. Moving to either side of the bed

e. Moving to head and foot of the bed

f. Performing pressure relief in bed

Considerations

1. ROM: normal ROM particularly important at:

   - shoulders
   - hips

2. Tone

3. Existing pressure sores and/or fragile skin (may make activity more difficult)

4. Age

5. Obesity

Process

1. Evaluate motor skills.

2. Evaluate functional component skills:

   - weight shift in lower developmental postures
   - balance and equilibrium reactions on elbows
   - compensatory movement patterns to compensate for absent musculature
   - skills to compensate for abnormal tone

3. Improve motor skills.

4. Teach functional component skills.

5. Determine appropriate bed mobility techniques.

6. Evaluate potential equipment needs.

7. Teach bed mobility skills.

8. Determine equipment needs.

9. Instruct nursing staff, OT, and significant others in patient's bed mobility skills.

10. Incorporate skills into daily routine.

11. Evaluate performance in daily routine.

12. Assist patient in problem solving to alleviate difficulties.

Pressure Relief

When sensation and motor control are intact, most patients will shift their weight around in a chair often enough to prevent the squeezing off of local blood supplies, which can create small areas of ischemia that will in turn quickly lead to pressure sores. However, the SCI patient with impaired sensation does not perceive the usual sensory cue to move and, in addition, often does not have the muscle power to move in the same way he did before. New habits and movement patterns must be developed to compensate for these losses.

ACHIEVING THE OUTCOME

Research indicates a correlation between the intensity and duration of pressure in pressure sore development. Clinical application of this research has led to the suggestion that pressure relief maneuvers be done every 10-15 minutes while sitting in a W/C to unweight the sitting surfaces, especially the ischial tuberosities since they are particularly prone to pressure sore development.

This fairly standard protocol is a time-consuming and tedious task. And, in fact, many patients just don't follow through with this suggestion. Interestingly enough, many of these same patients don't develop pressure sores. Why? Research has yet to give a satisfactory explanation for this clinical finding.

So, while this protocol may represent a good starting point, it may not necessarily be the desired end point. However, since the research labs have not given clear guidance in this area, the therapist is left with the task of individually evaluating the protocol with each patient.

Therapists have a professional obligation to start with the standard protocol. However, if the patient follows this procedure and the patient's skin remains in good condition, perhaps the time between pressure relief maneuvers should be slowly increased. It is likely that patient follow through would improve if this time between maneuvers could be increased.

As always, any changes in individual pressure relief protocol should be carefully monitored and well documented. Perhaps the time can be upgraded only on certain cushions or only at certain points in the treatment program when the patient's overall activity level increases. After all, essentially any movement within a W/C can act as a pressure relief maneuver. Perhaps this is one reason why the active patient can seemingly get by with fewer "formal" push-ups or leans. Relief occurs during the patient's transfers or during the shifting of weight in the chair to take a turn or when reaching for something from a shelf. Careful clinical observations can lead to a clearer understanding of pressure sore development and help streamline treatment programs in this area.

The following is a list of possible pressure relief maneuvers. It is, however, by no means an exhaustive list. As stated above, almost any movement can give pressure relief.

- Push-up. The patient places hands on both armrests or both wheels and lifts the buttocks off the seat.
- Forward lean. In the presence of trunk musculature, triceps, or strong anterior pectoral muscles, the patient flexes the trunk and leans his forearms on his thighs. In the absence of the above musculature or of sitting balance, he throws one arm over the W/C push handle and leans forward, reaching forward with the other arm.
- Side lean. The patient hooks one arm or wrist under the W/C push handles and leans over the opposite wheel. If he feels insecure, the W/C can be positioned beside a bed or another piece of furniture and that arm rest removed; he can then lean onto the furniture. Loops can be applied to the armrests and the arm secured in the loop, using biceps control to lean in the opposite direction.
- Mechanical alternative. A motorized recliner W/C can be used. When pressure relief is needed, the patient is able to recline the chair electrically. Various control systems are available.

EQUIPMENT OPTIONS

Cushions

With all the many cushions on the market, selecting the right one can be an overwhelming task. Many variables need to be considered: patient comfort, cushion durability and cost, patient function, and so on. Duration of pressure has already been discussed as a factor in pressure sore development. But, perhaps, before one can make an appropriate cushion selection, some of the other factors known to contribute to the development of pressure sores should be discussed.

Pressure

Arteriolar pressure in the skin capillaries is approximately 32 mm Hg. Many have believed that if the pressures under the patient's sitting surface could be kept below this level, pressure sores would not develop. Several different research projects have been conducted in an effort to find the cushion with the best contact pressure relief qualities. However, the results are confusing; no one seems to be able to agree on any one cushion. Perhaps some of the confusion is due to the fact that there were poor postural controls. Only recently have researchers and clinicians begun to seriously look at posture and realize the impact that asymmetries and poor postural alignment can have on pressure distribution and thus pressure sore development. (For more specifics on posture see Unit 9). In addition, although some cushions are reportedly quite good at decreasing surface pressure (notably the Roho and Jay cushions and some of the cut-out or molded foam cushions), no cushion on the market has been consistently able to maintain pressures below 32 mm Hg.

Shearing and Friction Forces

Although there appears to be a correlation between low contact pressure readings and the absence of pressure sores, low contact pressures are not the only thing to consider. Accurate measurement is often difficult to achieve. In addition, it should be noted that most techniques are only able to evaluate the static situation. Although it may be appropriate to place high priority on this factor with patients who have a more sedentary life style, it may be inappropriate to do this with more active patients. For these patients, shearing and friction forces may be a more important consideration.

When a patient is active, it is not uncommon for layers of tissue to be moving in opposite directions on the cushion. Blood supplies can again be cut off to tissue as blood vessels are stretched or angulated.

Horizontal stiffness is a term used by some researchers to measure a cushion's ability to compensate for shearing forces. Too much stiffness will not provide adequate compensation for these forces. Too little stiffness may have adverse effects on balance.

Some researchers believe that gel cushions are particularly effective in decreasing shearing forces. Even though these cushions may not provide the lowest contact pressures, they may be the cushion of choice for the more active patient.

Moisture

Moisture can also contribute to tissue maceration and damage. Many of the foams used in cushions are more porous and can therefore limit buildup of moisture. However, this advantage is often negated by less porous materials used to cover the foam. This can also be a limiting factor with many of the gel and flotation cushions that use plastic coverings. Even if these cushions are used, moisture buildup can be decreased by wearing cotton underwear, by using terry toweling or sheepskin over the cushion, or by simply increasing the frequency of push-ups.

Heat

If local temperatures are elevated, metabolism will increase and tissues will demand more oxygen even though the supply is already compromised. Foam cushions tend to increase local skin temperatures. Research indicates that heat will also increase when using flotation cushions, but this usually takes three to four hours of continuous use. Patients seem to confirm this, frequently reporting that they believe the Jobst cushions are cooler.

Choosing the Right Cushions

Knowing that no perfect cushion exists, how does the therapist decide which cushion is most appropriate? The key to this question can be found in looking at the patient and his life style needs. What are the priorities in his life?

If funding is an issue, the more expensive cushions, such as the Jay or the Roho cushions, might be eliminated.

Foam cushions often need to be replaced every 6 to 18 months. Roho cushions are easily punctured. Those patients especially concerned with durability would perhaps look at other cushions.

The patient himself can provide some clues as to which cushion might be most appropriate. Older patients tend to have lower skin capillary pressures. Some studies have measured this to be as low as 20 mm Hg. Thin and bony patients have less fat to cover bony prominences. Both of these patient groups may require cushions that will provide lower contact pressure relief.

Cushions that provide lower contact pressure relief may also be indicated for flaccid patients. As the thighs atrophy, the support area for sitting will be decreased, which will in turn increase the pressure under the ischial tuberosities.

Patients with sensation often find the contoured foam cushions uncomfortable.

If the patient is not bowel and bladder continent, cushions using less porous covers will have to be considered. Remember, however, that some coverings will take away from the inherent pressure relief qualities of the cushion material. Many of the plastic covers on the gel and flotation cushions, for instance, can produce a sling effect and do not allow the cushion material to

envelop the patient. Both of these effects tend to increase contact pressure.

Functional considerations are also important. An active patient who will be transferring in and out of the W/C into the car, onto a work bench, and so on may be more concerned with cushion weight. Gel cushions and Jobst cushions tend to be heavier (10 to 20 pounds) and therefore harder to move. Contoured cushions can make transfers more difficult. Patients sometimes have trouble lifting out of the ischial depression. Sitting balance is sometimes more difficult to achieve on Roho cushions. Transfers may also be harder using this cushion.

Careful consideration is essential to proper cushion selection. However it should be noted that none of the commercially available cushions seems able to control all the physical factors that have been noted in the literature to contribute to development of pressure sores. In addition, no cushion can ever hope to control the physiological and metabolic factors, such as protein deficiency, anemia, edema, and infection, which can also have a significant impact on development of pressure sores. Therefore, whether a patient develops a pressure sore may be largely determined by his behavior and the responsibility he assumes in caring for his body.

Mechanical Pressure Relief Options

Modern technology has created an electric W/C that can not only be electrically propelled but also can be electrically reclined. This provides even the very dependent quadriplegic patient with a means of independent pressure relief.

W/Cs will be discussed in more detail in later chapters, but it seems appropriate to discuss this particular W/C at this point. An extensive comparison of such sophisticated equipment is beyond the scope of this guide, but some general observations will be made.

There are basically three systems on the market today—the Duretech system sold through Abbey vendors, the Medicliner sold through the MED company, and the DO-IT system, sold through a company affiliated with Prentke-Romich. All three of these systems use an E&J recliner W/C as the base chair. Each chair has a little different look, but the engineering on each chair seems to be fairly comparable.

Both the Duretech and the Medicliner can be operated with almost any type of control—hand switches, breath control (sip and puff), chin control, and so on. The straw on the sip and puff control used with the Duretech chair is larger and perhaps less cosmetic than the one on the Medicliner. The Duretech straw is also quite flexible. If the straw gets too long, it may even have a tendency to migrate away from the user's mouth. On the other hand, the straw used with the Medicliner system will stay in place and not migrate from the user, but it is much more fragile; it tends to break easily.

The DO-IT system cannot be operated with a sip and puff control. This company's emphasis has been on chin controls. They have a very small and cosmetic chin control that fits on a collar harness that is worn around the patient's neck.

The Medicliner system can place the reclining unit on the back of the chair as well as under the seat. Placing the reclining unit on the W/C back can provide the added strength that might be needed to accommodate the stress of a large patient. On the other hand, if the reclining system is mounted on the back, there is very little space on the back frame to mount such things as BFOs and trunk supports. The reclining units of the Duretech and DO-IT systems can only be placed under the seat.

The DO-IT system seems to have more adjustability in the controls of the W/C. Not only can the forward acceleration and deceleration be adjusted, but the acceleration and deceleration of turns can also be separately adjusted. In addition, the trim can be adjusted to ensure that the chair moves in a straight line.

All three chairs will interface with almost any environmental control system; however, unless a rehabilitation engineering department is readily accessible, it is generally advisable to use the system each company sells with their chairs.

Durability is basically the same for all three chairs. For the most part the chairs are quite durable. However, because of the sophistication of this equipment, frequent repairs may be needed. Many patients advocate taking the chair in for a "check-up" every four months. Repairs should be done by the same company that sold the chair. If not, the warranty may not be valid.

Which chair is appropriate for a specific patient will again depend on the patient and his or her priorities. If he or she needs the sip and puff to control the chair, the DO-IT system is not an option. On the other hand, DO-IT has one of the nicest chin controls.

The argument against the chin control has always been cosmetic, primarily because the initial controls consisted of a large box that had to be placed in front of a patient's face for operation. The chin control, however, has the advantage of having proportional control. This allows the patient to more easily change speeds. While the sip and puff control may be more cosmetic, it does not have quite this much flexibility. One puff will start the chair and maintain it at a constant speed. A second puff is needed to increase the speed.

If the patient has a strong preference for a particular environmental control system, he should choose a W/C made by the same company. Because repairs are frequently needed, the W/C should probably be bought from the most accessible vendor.

No system is perfect for everyone. The patient should choose the system that meets his or her specific needs.

Pressure Relief—C4 Quadriplegic

Outcome

1. Patient demonstrates ability to perform independently pressure relief activities with motorized reclining W/C (will not be able to use upper extremities for controls).

2. Patient demonstrates ability to direct pressure relief and positioning in W/C.

Components

a. Relieving ischial pressure
b. Relieving sacral pressure
c. Relieving greater trochanter tuberosity pressure
d. Repositioning self after weight shift
e. Good body mechanics being included in directions to assistant

Considerations

1. Strength:

   • neck musculature
   • available movement patterns

2. ROM: Particularly important at:

   • trunk—lateral and forward flexion
   • hips

3. Respiratory status as it relates to ability to direct care

4. Immobilization devices and existing pressure sores or fragile skin may make activity more difficult.

5. Fear of falling out of W/C

6. Equipment: What is available to assist?

   • type of W/C
   • type of controls

7. Personality prior to injury:

   • how assertive was patient?

Process

1. Evaluate motor skills.

2. Evaluate functional component skills:

   • head control
   • comfort with being handled and moved
   • respiratory skills needed to direct care
   • manipulation of controls

3. Improve motor skills.

4. Teach functional component skills.

5. Evaluate potential equipment needs:

   • considering consultation with OT, Research and Engineering

6. Teach pressure relief skills:

   • teaching operation of controls on motorized W/C
   • practicing various methods of relief without electric W/C
     • side-to-side lean
     • forward lean

7. Instruct nursing staff, other team members, and significant others in patient's pressure relief skills.

8. Incorporate skills into daily routine.

9. Evaluate performance in daily routine.

10. Assist patient in problem solving to alleviate difficulties.

11. Determine appropriate equipment.

Pressure Relief—C5 Quadriplegic

Outcome

1. Patient demonstrates ability to perform independently pressure relief activities with motorized reclining W/C *with hand controls.*

2. Patient demonstrates ability to direct and/or *assist* with pressure relief activities and positioning in manual W/C.

Components

a. Relieving ischial pressure
b. Relieving sacral pressure
c. Relieving greater trochanter tuberosity pressure
d. Repositioning self after weight shift
e. Good body mechanics being included in directions to assistant

Considerations

1. Strength, especially:
   - *serratus anterior and scapular adductors*
   - *shoulder flexors and extensors*
   - *elbow flexors*

2. ROM:
   - *shoulder extension within normal limits*
   - trunk lateral and forward flexion
   - hip flex within normal limits

3. Tone *(particularly, increase in upper extremities)*

4. Respiratory status as it relates to ability to direct care

5. Existing pressure sores or fragile skin (may make activity more difficult)

6. *Fear of falling out of W/C*

7. Equipment: What is available to assist?
   - type of W/C, controls, adaptations
   - *cushions provide varying degrees of relief*
   - *adjustable armrests (can make the activity easier)*

8. Personality prior to injury:
   - how assertive was patient?

Process

1. Evaluate motor skills.

2. Evaluate functional component skills:
   - head control
   - comfort with being handled and moved
   - manipulation of controls
   - respiratory skills needed to direct care
   - *weight shift in sitting and on elbows*
   - *compensatory movement patterns to compensate for absent musculature*
   - *compensatory sensory techniques*
   - *skills to compensate for abnormal tone*

3. Improve motor skills.

4. Teach functional component skills.

5. Evaluate potential equipment needs.

6. Teach pressure relief skills:
   - teaching operation of controls on motorized W/C
   - teaching various methods of relief without electric W/C
     - side-to-side lean
     - *forward flexion*
     - *forward flexion with rotation*
     - *use of arm loops*
     - *hooking arms behind push handles*

7. Instruct nursing staff, other team members, and significant others in patient's pressure relief skills.

8. Incorporate skills into daily routine.

9. Evaluate performance in daily routine.

10. Assist patient in problem solving to alleviate difficulties.

11. Determine appropriate equipment.

Pressure Relief—C6 Quadriplegic

Outcome

Patient demonstrates ability to perform independently all pressure relief and repositioning in W/C.

Components

a. Relieving ischial pressure
b. Relieving sacral pressure
c. Relieving greater trochanter tuberosity pressure
d. Repositioning self after weight shift

Considerations

1. Strength, especially:

    - *shoulder depressors*
    - shoulder flexion and extension
    - shoulder adductors
    - elbow flexors
    - *wrist extensors*

2. ROM:

    - shoulder extension within normal limits
    - *elbow extension within normal limits*
    - *wrist within normal limits*
    - hip flexion within normal limits

3. Tone

4. Fear of falling out of W/C

5. *Age*

6. *Obesity*

7. Equipment: What is available?

    - type of cushion (Some provide more relief than others.)
    - *loops, adjustable armrests, etc.*

Process

1. Evaluate motor skills.

2. Evaluate functional component skills:

    - weight shift on elbows *and with extended arms in sitting*
    - *balance and equilibrium reaction on elbows and with extended arms in sitting, as well as without upper-extremity support*
    - compensatory sensory techniques
    - skills to compensate for abnormal tone

3. Improve motor skills.

4. Teach functional component skills.

5. Evaluate potential equipment needs.

6. Teach pressure relief skills, providing as many options as possible:

    - side-to-side lean
    - forward flexion with rotation
    - *½ push-up with elbows on raised armrests*
    - *½ push-up on locked elbows with hands on tires (placing 1 arm behind the push handle may facilitate this)*

7. Instruct nursing staff, other team members, and significant others in patient's pressure relief skills.

8. Incorporate skills into daily routine.

9. Assist patient in problem solving to alleviate difficulties.

10. Determine appropriate equipment.

Pressure Relief—C7–8 Quadriplegic

Outcome

Patient demonstrates ability to independently perform all pressure relief and repositioning in W/C *(including W/C push-ups)*.

Components

a. Relieving ischial pressure
b. Relieving sacral pressure
c. Relieving greater trochanter tuberosity pressure
d. Repositioning self after weight shift

Considerations

1. Strength, especially:

   • shoulder depressors
   • *triceps*
   • entire upper extremities

2. ROM, especially:

   • hip flexion to at least 90°
   • elbow extension within normal limits

3. Tone

4. Obesity

5. Age

6. Equipment: What is available to assist?

   • cushions
   • adjustable armrests

Process

1. Evaluate motor skills.

2. Evaluate functional component skills:

   • balance and equilibrium reactions in sitting with and without upper extremity support
   • *ability to lift body weight on extended elbows*
   • skills to compensate for abnormal tone

3. Improve motor skills.

4. Teach functional component skills.

5. Evaluate potential equipment needs.

6. Teach pressure relief:

   • *patient will generally use push-up.*

7. Instruct nursing staff, other team members, and significant others in patient's pressure relief skills.

8. Incorporate skills into daily routine.

9. Evaluate performance in daily routine.

10. Assist patient in problem solving to alleviate difficulties.

11. Determine appropriate equipment.

Pressure Relief—Paraplegic

Outcome

Patient demonstrates ability to independently perform all pressure relief and repositioning in W/C including W/C push-ups.

Components

a.   Relieving ischial pressure
b.   Relieving sacral pressure
c.   Relieving greater trochanter tuberosity pressure
d.   Repositioning self after weight shift

Considerations

1. ROM, especially:

   - hip flexion to at least 90°
   - elbow extension within normal limits

2. Tone

3. Obesity

4. Age

5. Equipment: What is available to assist?

   - cushions
   - adjustable armrests

Process

1. Evaluate motor skills.

2. Evaluate functional component skills:

   - balance and equilibrium reactions with and without upper extremity support
   - ability to lift body weight on extended elbows
   - skills to compensate for abnormal tone

3. Improve motor skills.

4. Teach functional component skills.

5. Evaluate potential equipment needs.

6. Teach pressure relief skills:

   - patient will generally use push-up

7. Instruct nursing staff, other team members, and significant others in patient's pressure relief skills.

8. Incorporate into daily routine.

9. Evaluate performance in daily routine.

10. Assist patient in problem solving to alleviate difficulties.

11. Determine appropriate equipment.

Transfers

Most SCI patients can no longer stand up and walk to the next chair or into the bathroom. Moving from one surface to the next becomes a major task with all kinds of steps—placing the sliding board, positioning the legs, managing the W/C—in addition to the actual move to and from a surface. How can this whole process be accomplished?

ACHIEVING THE OUTCOME

Bed Transfers

Bed transfers are often the first transfers taught. All other transfers will build on the skills that are developed here.

Firmer surfaces are usually easier to learn on, and so a mat is frequently used in initial training. After the patient has achieved some measure of success with transfers to and from a mat, training is then moved to the bed.

Transfers are usually taught in steps. A patient may spend a month learning all the component parts (e.g., placing the board, managing the legs, moving to and from the W/C) of a transfer before he puts it all together in one sequence. Each of the component parts will require varying amounts of skill in the use of such things as rotation, weight shifts, and balance. Where one

starts in this transfer training process will depend on what functional skills each patient begins with. Different approaches to the various component parts of the transfer are presented on the following pages. Some require more balance in sitting; others require more balance on elbows. Some require more ROM; others require more strength. Again, how the various approaches to the different transfer components are combined will depend on the patient and his skills.

It is important to note that the more approaches the patient is able to use the more independent he will be. He will more likely be able to deal with any situation that arises. Therefore, after the patient finds one approach that works for him, he should be encouraged to experiment and develop other methods.

Transfer training should be a problem-solving activity for both the therapist and the patient. Much experimentation is required to develop the best transfer for each individual. Each patient will develop his own special way of transferring. For this reason, it would be impossible to list all the possible approaches. The ideas presented are meant to be starting points in this problem-solving process; only a few of the many options are presented.

Finally, it should be remembered that with increased deficits in strength, moving on and off different surfaces will be time consuming and require much energy. A quadriplegic patient may spend as long as 20 minutes

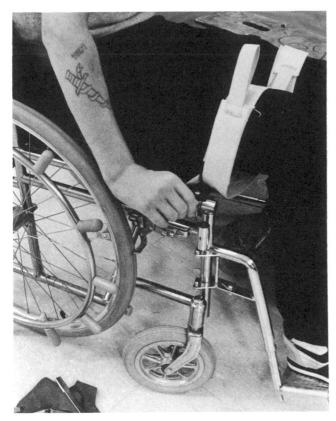

Figure 8–1a Locking brakes

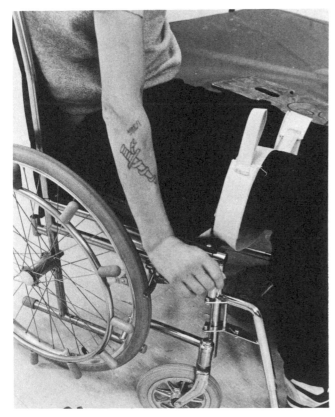

Figure 8–1b

to complete initial transfers. It will therefore be essential to develop a transfer that will require as few steps as possible. Each step will cost more time and energy. Speed is gained not only as the patient learns to move faster and acquires the endurance needed to work for longer periods without rest but also as he is able to cut out steps from the process.

Management of W/C Parts

Brakes. With wrist extensors, locking and unlocking the W/C can usually be accomplished quite easily (Figures 8–1a and 8–1b). Brake extensions may also be considered. These are easier to reach and require less trunk balance. The longer lever arm facilitates easy locking. However, since they need to be removed before getting out of the W/C, they add another step to the whole process of transferring and are, in addition, another item to lose.

One possible approach to locking the W/C in the presence of weak or absent wrist extensors would be to have loops attached to a splint. These can then be hooked onto the brakes to lock and unlock them (Figure 8–2). This approach will again add more steps to the transfer. The patient now has to put on the splint to lock the W/C. In addition, the splint may interfere with other aspects of the transfer and then need to be removed.

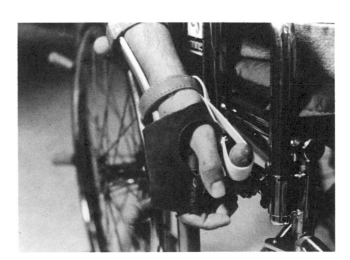

Figure 8–2 Locking brakes c̄ loop

Foot Pedals. Because of sensory deficits and general unfamiliarity with the W/C itself, patients often have some initial trouble finding the lever to push that will release the pedal. A variety of approaches can be used. Those with wrist extensors can lean over the side and use the back of their hand (Figures 8–3a and 8–3b) or the palm of their hand to push the lever around. Others, who are more comfortable leaning forward, choose to reach under their legs and use their tight finger or thumb muscles to pull the lever until it releases. From this position the lever may be easier to see.

Some patients consider having quad releases put on the lever. Unlocking the foot pedals becomes easier, but the pedals are then much more difficult to reattach to the W/C if they need to be removed.

Elevating legrests should be avoided. These usually need to be taken off (not just swung away) before the transfer. They are heavier and more awkward to both remove and reattach.

How a pedal reattaches to the W/C often depends on which company made it. Most companies make pedals that have to be attached to the side of the W/C and then swung around in place. Others have pedals that will attach with the pedal in the front of the W/C. This avoids the extra step of moving away from the bed to make room for the pedal. All pedals will automatically lock once swung into place.

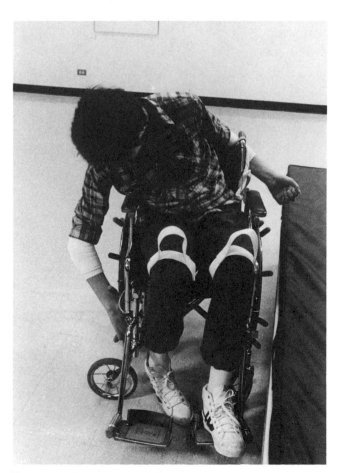

Figure 8–3a Removing foot pedals

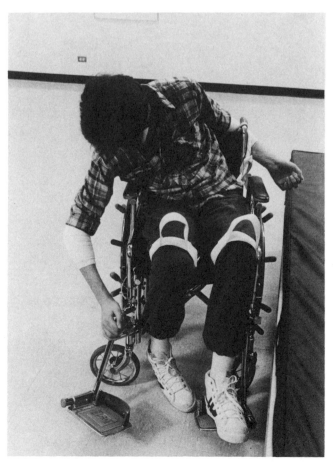

Figure 8–3b

Side Panel. In the presence of weak or absent hand musculature, side panels can easily be locked and unlocked with a quad release, which is a flat button that pushes the pin out of the hole that locks the armrest into place.

The actual removal of the side panel can be a little more difficult and usually requires some finesse. The front and back struts of the panel need to be lifted out evenly. With wrist extensors or hand musculature, this is done fairly easily (Figures 8–4a and 8–4b). Without wrist extensors the panel can still be removed using the biceps. The patient will just need to make sure that he is lifting from the center of the panel.

After removing the panel, it should be put in a place where it can easily be reached when it needs to be re-attached. Reattaching the panel is often a more complicated task than removal because of sensory deficits and the difficulties in seeing where the struts of the panel fit. Wraparound armrests can be even more difficult to reattach because the back strut fits into a hole behind the W/C back frame.

Sliding Board Placement

Placement of the sliding board should be approximately mid thigh (Figure 8–5). If it is too close to the

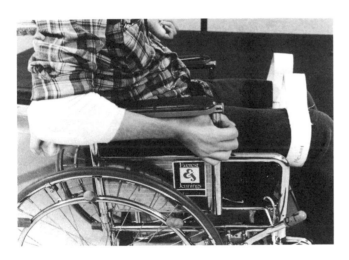

Figure 8–4a Removal of side panel

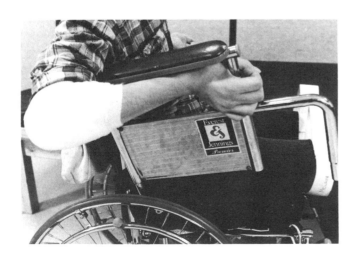

Figure 8–4b

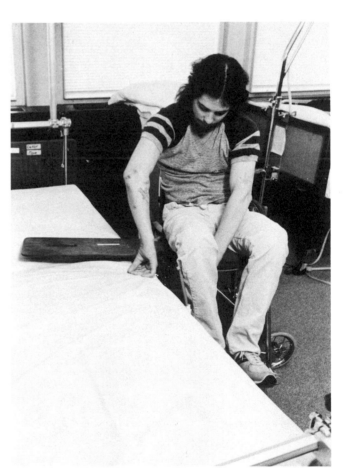

Figure 8–5 Sliding board placement should be at the mid-thigh level.

knee, the slide will be more difficult. If it is too far back, the patient may slide forward off the board.

Many different types of sliding boards exist. When choosing a board, one of the things to determine is how the patient will "grip" the board and develop enough traction to push it under his seat. Some patients prefer a board made with a hole that they can then hook into with their tight finger flexors (Figure 8–6). Others seem able to use a smooth board with no holes (Figure 8–7). These patients, however, may choose to use a

palm glove, which will provide some resistance on the board as they push it under the seat (Figure 8–8).

Attaching loops to a board has also been considered. Some patients do find that they can hook into these loops and then use wrist extensors or biceps to position the board; however, the loops are often awkward to use. If loops are used, careful attachment is necessary. The attachments should not protrude to the other side because this may cause skin problems.

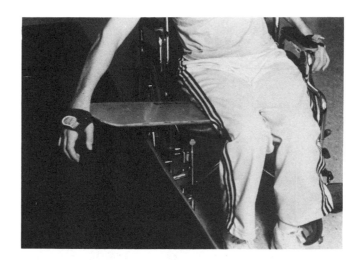

Figure 8–7 Sliding board is placed using edge of board to push under buttock.

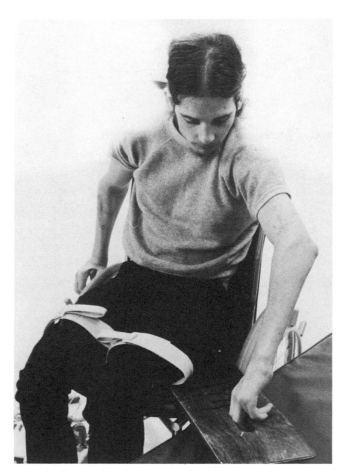

Figure 8–6 Sliding board is placed by hooking tight finger flexors into hole in board.

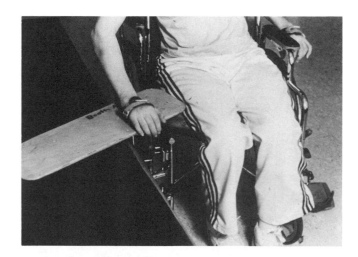

Figure 8–8 Sliding board is placed using resistance of palm glove to push board under buttocks.

Telescoping boards can also be used (Figures 8–9a through 8–9e). These boards are made with a telescoping tube attached to the back that fits into the hole where the front strut of the W/C side panel would ordinarily fit. Placement of these boards is easier, and patients are more secure in the fact that the board will not move. However, there is relatively little board under the seat of the patient in the W/C, which makes the slide across the cushion more difficult.

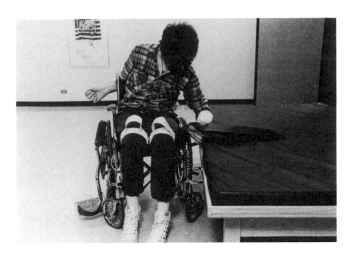

Figure 8–9a A telescoping sliding board can be used.

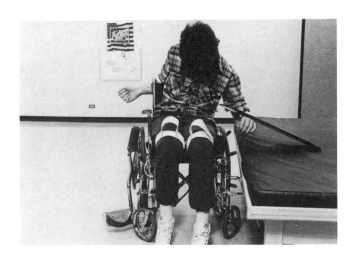

Figure 8–9b

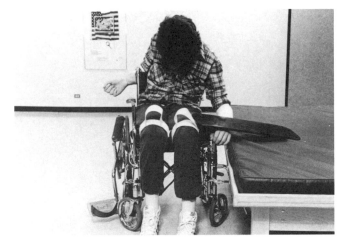

Figure 8–9c

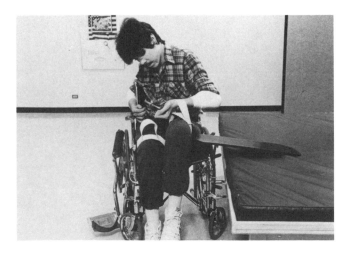

Figure 8–9d

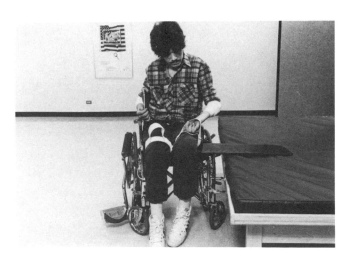

Figure 8–9e

Sometimes a patient is not able to wiggle and push the sliding board underneath his seat. This is especially difficult if a Roho cushion is used. Figures 8–10a through 8–10d show a patient who crosses her legs in order to get board placement. The actual placement can be done more easily; but this method does require more strength and power than those methods shown previously in which leverage, weight-shifting ability, and body mechanics seem to be the more important issues.

There are instances in which placement is only a matter of finesse (Figures 8–11a through 8–11f). The trick to this approach is found in the initial placement of the board on the hips. A little experimentation is usually needed to find the right spot. Successful placement using this method will require good bed mobility skills.

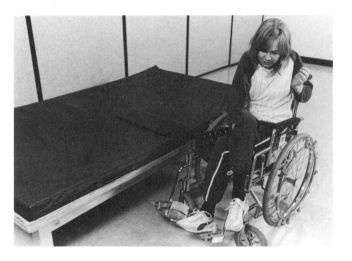

Figure 8–10a Legs are crossed to place sliding board.

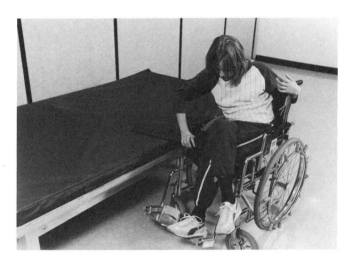

Figure 8–10b

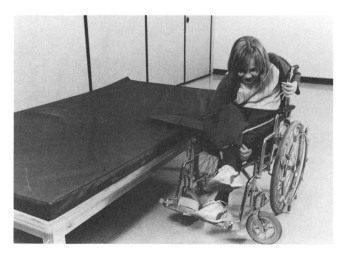

Figure 8–10c

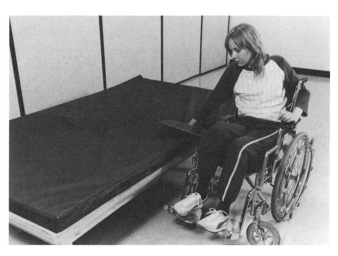

Figure 8–10d

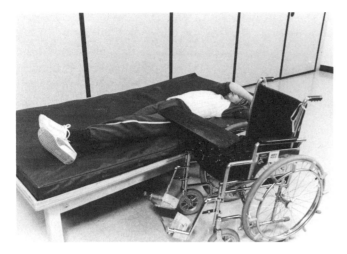

Figure 8–11a Rolling is used to assist in sliding board placement.

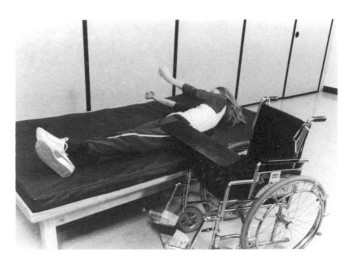

Figure 8–11b

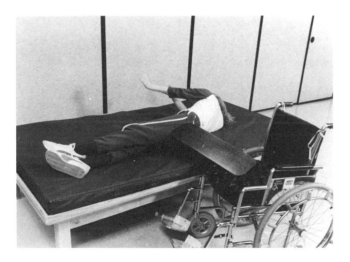

Figure 8–11c

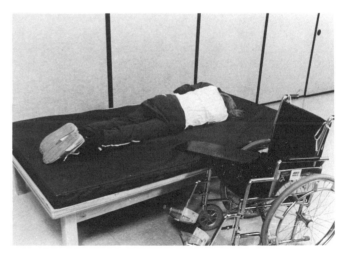

Figure 8–11d

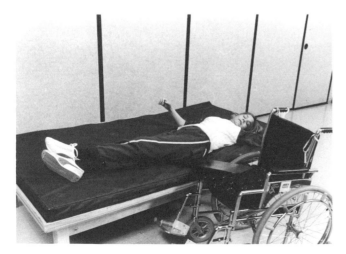

Figure 8–11e

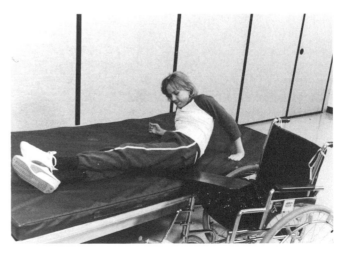

Figure 8–11f

If all else fails, be creative. The sliding board does not always have to go between the cushion and the patient. If the patient is only using the board as a bridge and not to help facilitate the slide, it may be easier to place the board underneath the cushion, especially if it is a Roho (Figure 8–12).

Removing the board is usually just a matter of shifting weight off the board and wiggling it out of place.

Clearing the Wheel

If the patient is unable to lift up and over the wheel, he will have to find some other way to clear the wheel. This can be done either before or after sliding board placement, depending on the patient and how he accomplishes other aspects of the transfer.

For some this is done most easily by arching the back and leaning into extension (Figure 8–13). Some increases in tone can facilitate this move; however, the patient needs to be able to control the tone. If not, he could possibly set off a full body extensor pattern that would push him out the front of the W/C. In any case, whether tone is present or not, the patient will still need to develop a good sense of where he is in space to know when to stop sliding forward.

This method is difficult to use in W/Cs with low back heights. In addition, it may not be the method of choice if the patient is unable to reposition himself for the rest of the transfer after he moves his hips forward.

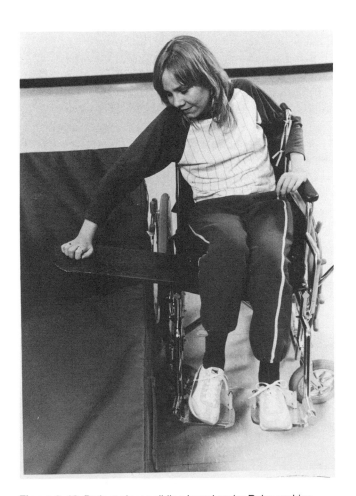

Figure 8–12 Patient places sliding board under Roho cushion.

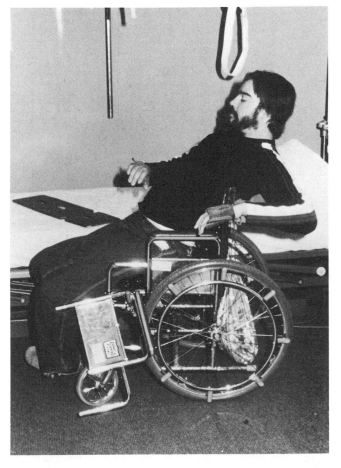

Figure 8–13 Patient is leaning back into extension to move hips forward and clear wheel.

Other methods of clearing the wheel can be used. To move the right hip forward, the left arm is hooked behind the left push handle and the right arm is swung forward and to the left across the chest. The left hip can be moved forward by repeating the above procedure.

The patient in Figure 8–14, in order to clear the wheel on the right, is using a similar but more exaggerated motion created by the momentum of falling forward and to the left. In addition to falling forward, the patient is also pulling with her left arm against the left push handle. The movement can also be accomplished by simultaneously pushing against the back wheel with the left hand and pulling against the left side panel with the right wrist extensor while falling forward and to the left. This procedure can initially be frightening but, if mastered, can be used to clear the wheel and, in addition, will often propel the patient one third of the way out of the wheelchair with minimal muscular effort. *Note:* Variations of these movement patterns can also be used by the patient to reposition himself in the W/C.

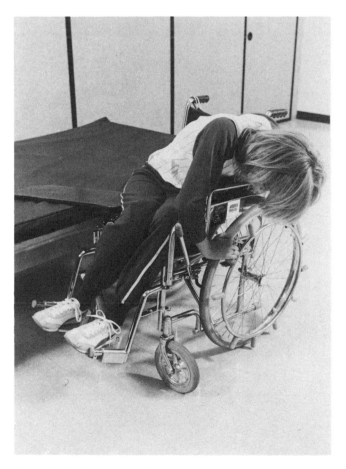

Figure 8–14 Patient uses the body mechanics of momentum and simple levers to clear the wheel.

Moving To and From the W/C

The SCI patient with hip and knee strength or increased lower extremity tone may be able to perform a stand-pivot transfer. This will require a certain degree of trunk balance and the ability to bear weight on at least one lower extremity.

If a patient is unable to do a stand-pivot transfer but is able to maintain straight arms via triceps or some other means of elbow locking and is able to achieve a functional lift, moving to and from the W/C can still be a fairly simple task. A lateral transfer may then be used (Figures 8–15a through 8–15c). It can be accomplished either with or without a sliding board.

This transfer requires good scapular depression (especially if done without a board), fair to good trunk balance in sitting, and a minimum of 90 degrees of hip flexion. Body proportions can also become a significant factor. Patients with relatively short arms may have more difficulty achieving a high enough lift.

The patient in Figure 8–15a is lifting on his knuckles. This can help facilitate a higher lift but probably should not be encouraged since the position requires that the force of the lift pass through the wrist. This can lead to capsulitis and other problems at the wrist.

Some patients are able to maintain elbow locking well but are unable to achieve a functional lift because of strength deficits and/or excessive ROM in the back and poor sitting balance. The patient in Figures 8–16a through 8–16c is using a little body mechanics and physics to move onto the mat. He has enough hip ROM to lean forward over his knees and away from the direction in which he wants to move. This means that he has less weight behind him to move and enables him to slide out of the W/C. Note the angle of his arms and the push. Most of the force is in a horizontal direction, not vertical as is seen in Figure 8–15b, in which the force was being used to develop a lift rather than a slide. Also note the palm gloves used by the patient in Figure 8–16a to help create traction between his hand and the pushing surface. Licking the palm of the hand can do the same thing.

This transfer may be more easily accomplished with a "wiggle." Rotating the shoulders will rock the hips, decreasing some of the inertia that is always present at the beginning of the movement, and make the push to and from the W/C easier.

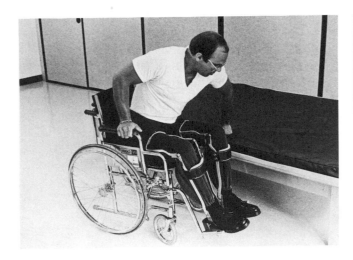

Figure 8–15a Lateral transfer

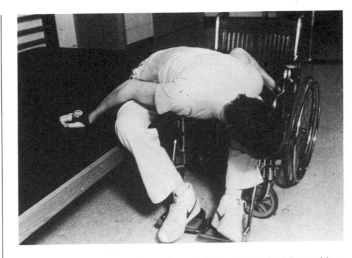

Figure 8–16a Patient performs lateral slide out of W/C while pushing with extended arms.

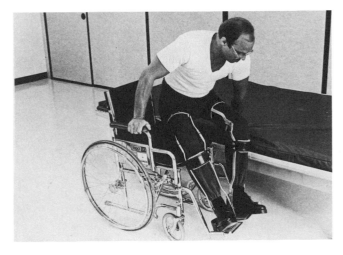

Figure 8–15b

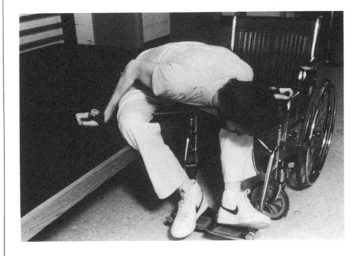

Figure 8–16b

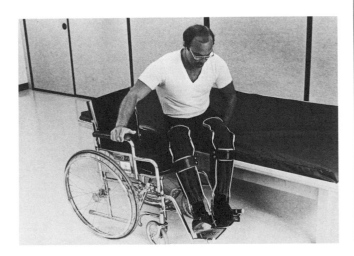

Figure 8–15c

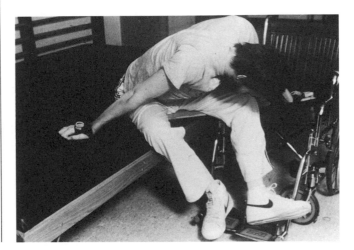

Figure 8–16c

The patient who has difficulty maintaining locked elbows may be able to transfer using a prone-on-elbows position (Figures 8–17a through 8–17c). In addition to a lot of energy and endurance, this transfer requires good hip and shoulder flexion as well as good scapular and shoulder stabilization. The need for good balance skills in the prone-on-elbows position should be readily apparent. After each push the patient will need to reposition his elbows; thus he needs to develop skill with controlled mobility and static-dynamic activities.

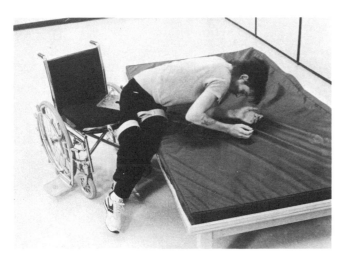

Figure 8–17a Patient uses prone-on-elbows push to slide back into W/C.

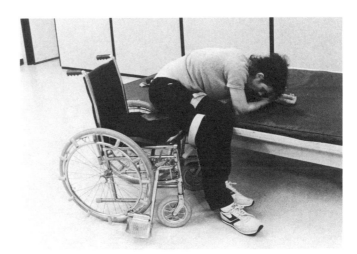

Figure 8–17b

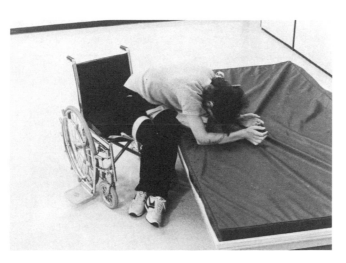

Figure 8–17c

A modified prone-on-elbows position can also be used to transfer out of the W/C (Figures 8–18a through 8–18c). Pushing out of the W/C in this manner requires many of the same skills required to push into the W/C seen in the sequence in Figures 8–17a through 8–17c.

Much of the success of this transfer is dependent on finding the right place from which to push off. Any number of different ways can be found. Much experimentation will need to occur before the right combination is found. The patient should focus on finding spots on the frame rather than on the chair upholstery to push on. This will prevent wear and tear of the upholstery.

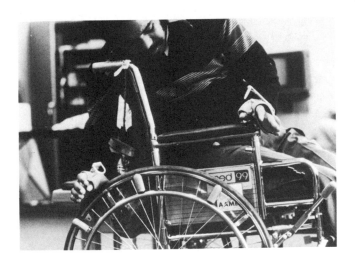

Figure 8–18a Patient uses modified prone-on-elbows push to transfer from W/C.

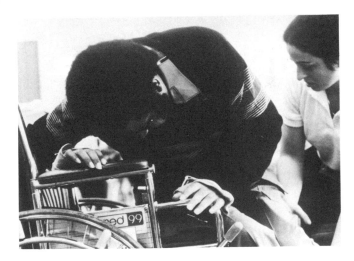

Figure 8–18b

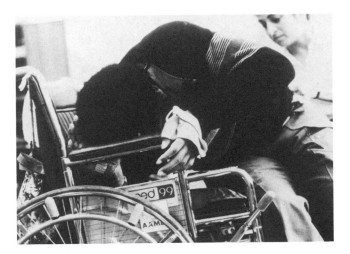

Figure 8–18c

There are times when there just does not seem to be a right spot on the W/C to use. The patient in Figures 8–19a and 8–19b hooks his arm under his legs and uses this position as a counterforce for the other arm to push against rather than using another spot on the W/C.

The head can be used to stabilize the trunk while one arm is being repositioned (Figures 8–20a and 8–20b). This can also provide the patient with a resting point, giving him time to collect the energy he will need for the next push.

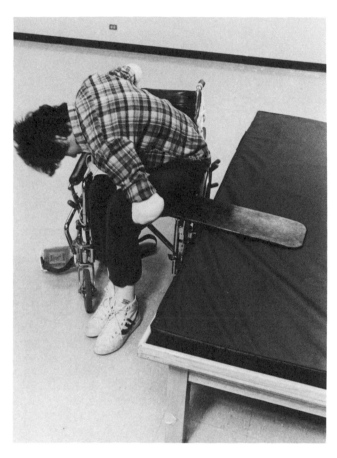

Figure 8–19a Patient hooks arm under leg to transfer from W/C.

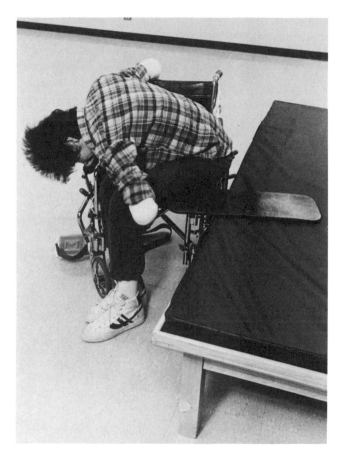

Figure 8–19b

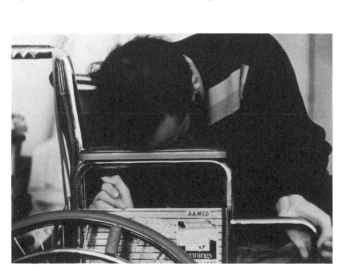

Figure 8–20a Patient uses head to stabilize trunk while repositioning arm.

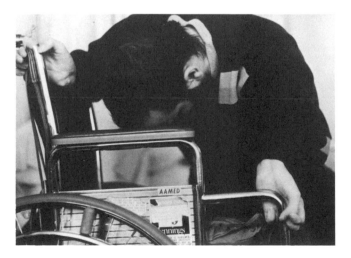

Figure 8–20b

The need for good coordination and body sense is readily apparent, particularly in light of the fact that many sensory modalities are usually impaired to some degree. In addition, vision can be blocked during many points in the transfer. The therapist may initially need to act as a substitute for the patient's poor sensory feedback systems, telling him where he is in space, until he develops his own alternative cues.

Short sitting does not have to be used as the starting position. Long sitting can also be used (Figures 8–21a through 8–21d). This position can often provide the patient some additional stability. Again, note the ROM requirements.

This method is usually easier to accomplish moving into the W/C than it is moving out of the W/C. When moving into the W/C the weight is forward and away from the direction of movement. Pushing is usually easier than pulling. When moving out of the W/C, much of the patient's weight is forward and in the direction of movement.

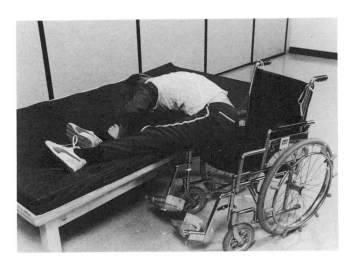

Figure 8–21a Patient slides into W/C from a long sitting position.

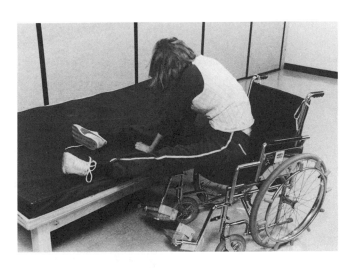

Figure 8–21b

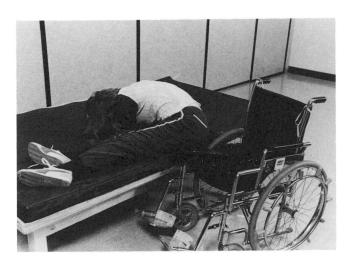

Figure 8–21c

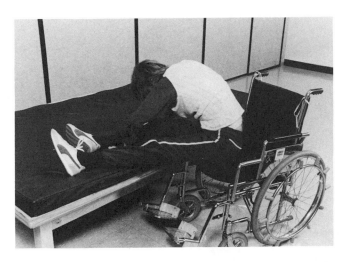

Figure 8–21d

The patient who needs to bring his legs up to the bed before beginning the slide out of the W/C, but is unable to pull out of the chair from a long sitting position, may be able to "roll out" of his chair (Figures 8–22a through 8–22c). The patient swings his arms to develop the momentum he needs to throw his trunk onto the bed (*Note:* This is often frightening initially). The actual move onto the bed requires very little muscular strength but the patient must have good bed mobility skills in order to reposition himself on the bed once there.

It is difficult at times to clear a 24-inch wheel, but this can be done if the patient first scoots forward in the chair and is able to develop good momentum with his swing.

Finally, there are times when the best transfer the patient is able to do seems to defy all logic of body mechanics. The patient in Figures 8–23a through 8–23d transfers most easily by pulling out of his W/C with his weight in the direction of the movement. Therefore, flexibility in this problem-solving process must be allowed for the seemingly impractical approach.

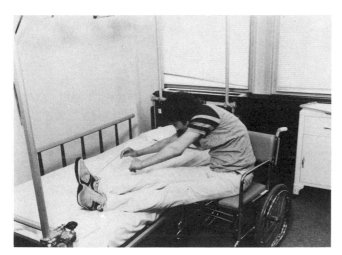

Figure 8–22a Patient "rolls" out of W/C.

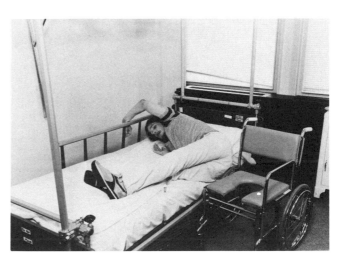

Figure 8–22b

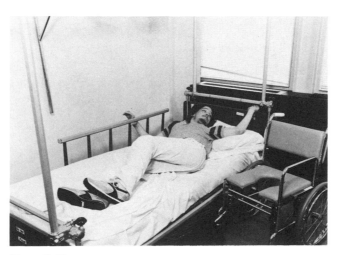

Figure 8–22c

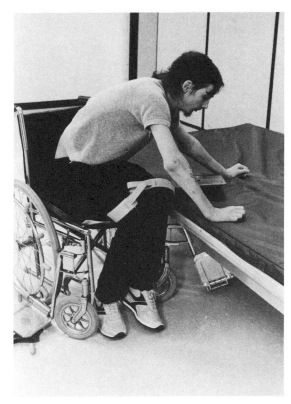

Figure 8–23a Patient places his weight in the direction of movement to transfer from W/C.

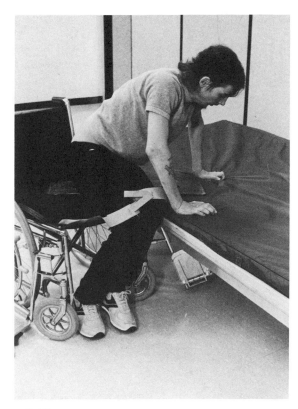

Figure 8–23b

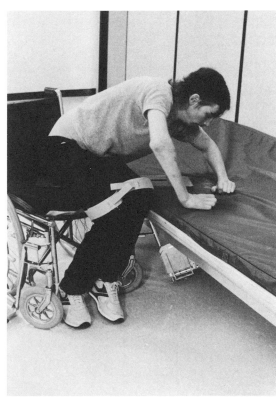

Figure 8–23c

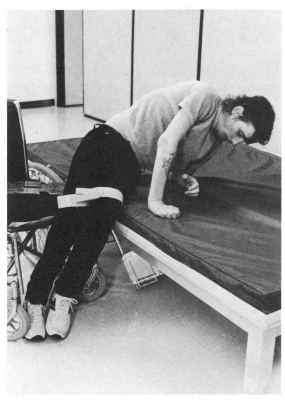

Figure 8–23d

Assuming a Stable Position

After moving to or from a W/C, the patient must be able to regain a stable position. With some trunk rotation and shoulder extension, the patient who has completed a move into the W/C will be able to throw his arm and hook it behind the W/C push handle. He can then use his wrist extensors and biceps to pull into sitting (Figures 8–24a and 8–24b).

If the patient is on the bed rather than in the W/C, a similar motion can be used. The patient hooks his wrist around his leg and again uses the wrist extensor and biceps to pull up to sitting (Figures 8–25a and 8–25b).

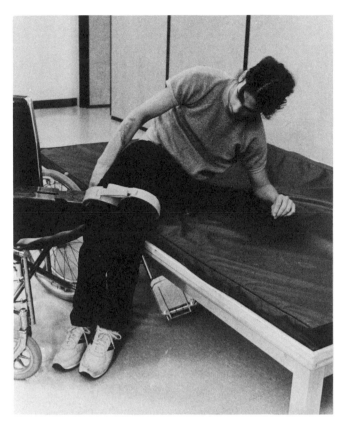

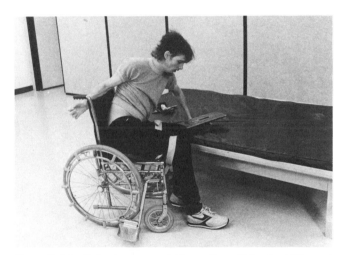

Figure 8–24a Patient assumes stable position with trunk rotation and shoulder extension by throwing his arm behind the W/C handle.

Figure 8–25a Patient hooks wrist around leg and uses wrist extensor and biceps to pull up to sitting position.

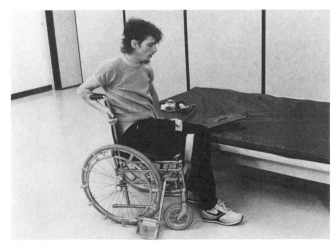

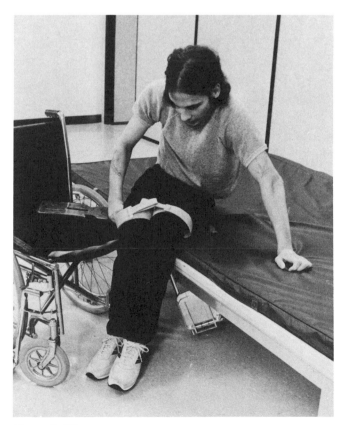

Figure 8–24b

Figure 8–25b

The pectoralis muscle in the opposite arm will assist the movement by pulling the arm into elbow extension. If the patient has difficulty developing enough strength, rocking back and forth on the elbow along with exaggerated head movements can make the activity easier.

With strong pectoralis muscles, a patient may be able to push straight up into sitting once on the mat (Figures 8–26a through 8–26d). The patient will need to exaggerate the external rotation at the shoulder to place the pectoralis musculature at its best mechanical advantage for elbow locking. Exaggerated head extension will also facilitate this process.

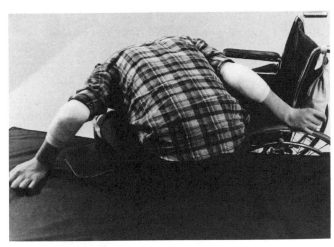

Figure 8–26a Patient uses pectoralis major and other arm muscles to push into sitting position. External rotation at the shoulder is exaggerated to facilitate the movement.

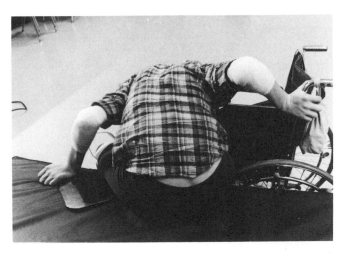

Figure 8–26b

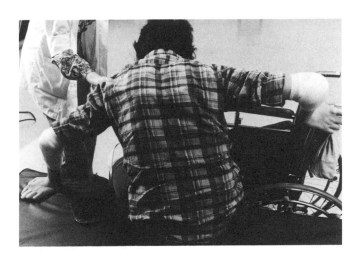

Figure 8–26c

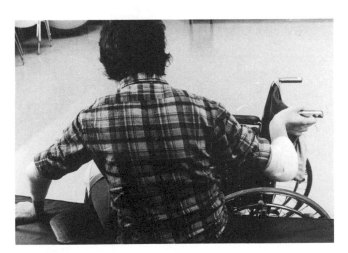

Figure 8–26d

For some patients, assuming sitting is just too difficult. However, they are still able to find a stable position on their elbows. The patient in Figures 8–27a through 8–27c places her left elbow back on the mat and pushes with her right arm until she is able to fall back on the left elbow. Head extension can again assist the movement. Good scapular and shoulder stabilization is needed.

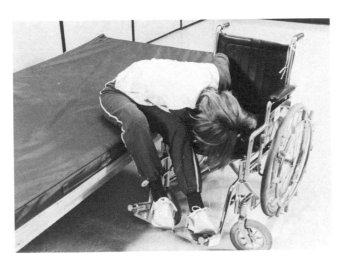

Figure 8–27a Patient assumes stable position by pushing back onto one elbow.

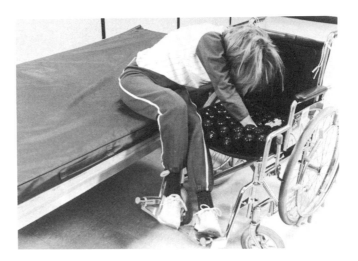

Figure 8–27b

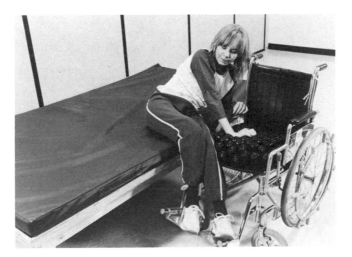

Figure 8–27c

Lower Extremity Management

One of the first times that skill in managing lower extremities is needed in the transfer procedure is in getting the feet off the foot pedals. Some patients use loops (Figure 8–28). Others use their biceps or wrist extensors (Figure 8–29) or hand musculature, if present, to hook under the leg and lift it up. If trunk balance is poor, the patient may also need to use one arm to stabilize the trunk.

Loops make the whole process easier but putting them on will add additional steps to the transfer and they are easily misplaced and lost. As patients develop more strength and skill, many will find that they no longer need this step.

Getting the feet back on the pedals is usually just a matter of reversing the procedure used to take them off.

Note: The feet do not have to be taken off the pedals. Some believe that this is a waste of time. However, those patients with increased flexor tone often find that their feet get tangled up in the pedals and then they have a harder time getting their legs onto the bed. Removing the pedals and putting the feet flat on the ground also seems to provide a firmer base of support.

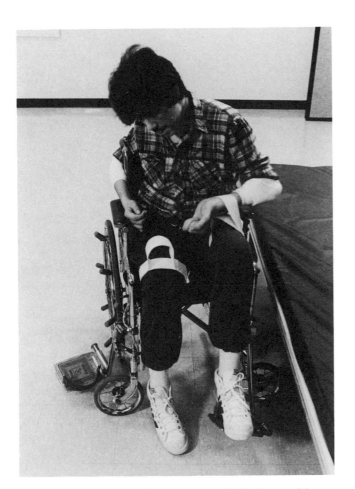

Figure 8–28 Patient uses a loop to remove his leg from pedal.

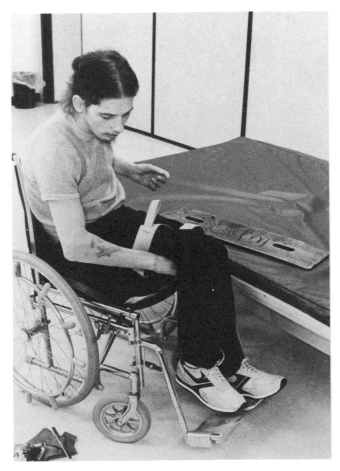

Figure 8–29 Patient uses wrist extensors to remove his leg from pedal.

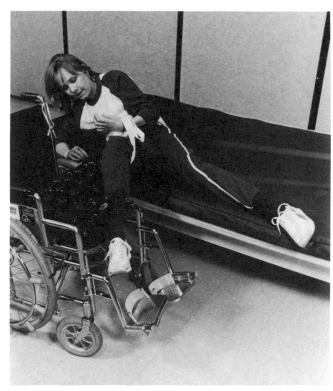

Figure 8–30a Patient uses a modified supine-on-elbows position to bring legs onto mat.

With deficits in both lower extremity and upper extremity strength as well as in trunk balance, getting the legs onto the bed can prove to be a real challenge. The patient in Figures 8–30a through 8–30c uses a modified supine-on-elbows position as a starting position. While balancing on one elbow she uses her biceps (wrist extensors can also be used) to hook into a loop and pulls her legs up one at a time. If a little flexion tone is present, the second leg will frequently come up on its own as the first leg is lifted up.

The prone-on-elbows position can also be used as a starting position. Note how much ROM and flexibility are used by the patient who chooses to use this approach (Figures 8–31a through 8–31h).

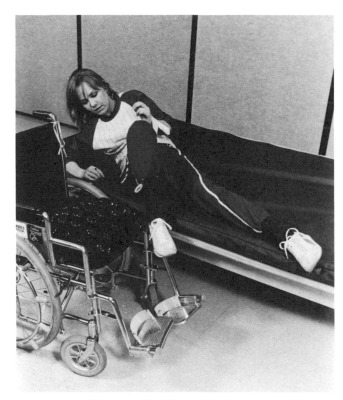

Figure 8–30b

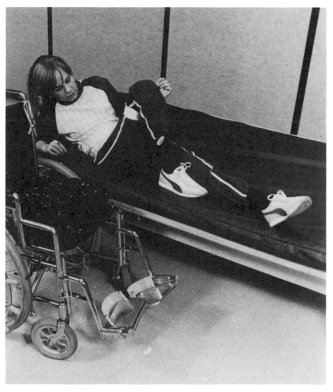

Figure 8–30c

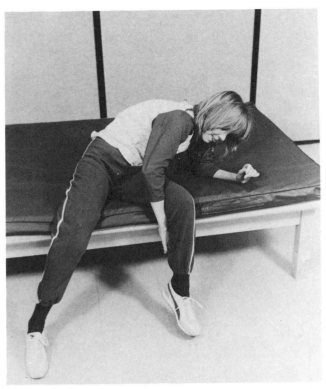

Figure 8–31a Patient uses prone-on-elbows position to manage her lower extremities. Note ROM and flexibility.

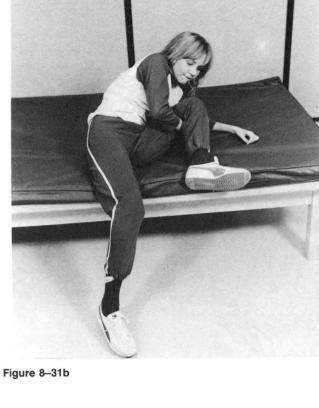

Figure 8–31b

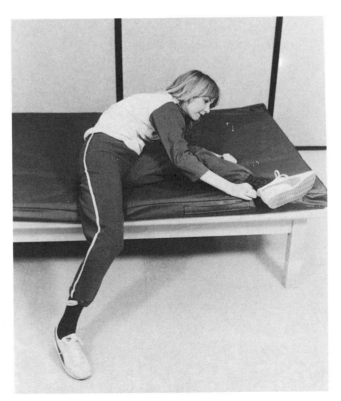

Figure 8–31c

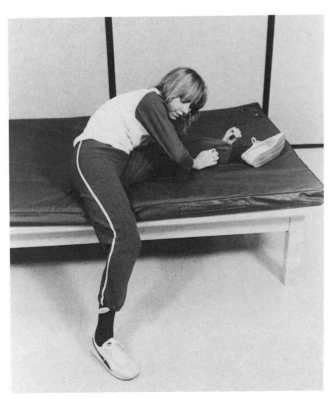

Figure 8–31d The patient will have to experiment with how far to push the first leg up. The leg will fall off if it is not on the mat well. If it is too far on the mat, the patient will be unable to reach the second leg.

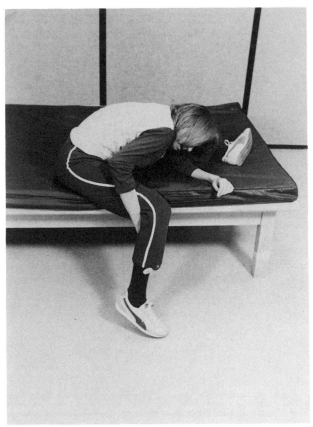

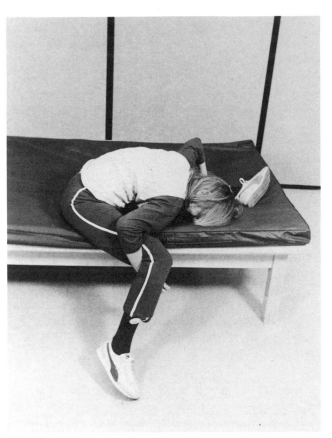

Figure 8–31e Note how the patient repositions her elbow in front of the leg. This allows her to reach the second leg and will provide her with some added stability as her arm braces against the leg.

Figure 8–31f

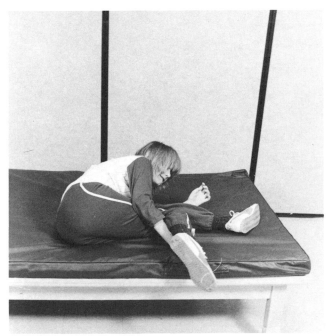

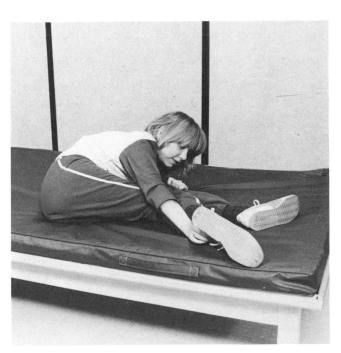

Figure 8–31g

Figure 8–31h

Several approaches can be taken from a sitting position. Loops can again be used, either around both legs together or around each individual leg. In this method the patient uses the momentum of his body falling backward as the power to pull his legs up. The patient in Figures 8–32a through 8–32c had particularly good sitting balance and so was able to use both arms hooked into individual loops. Some, however, need to use one arm extended behind them on the mat to stabilize the trunk while they position the other arm in the loop and initiate the rocking that is sometimes needed to throw the trunk back.

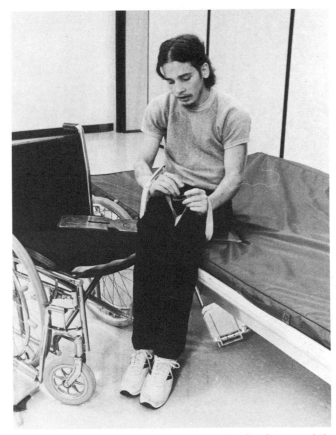

Figure 8–32a Patient moves legs onto mat using loops and the momentum of his body.

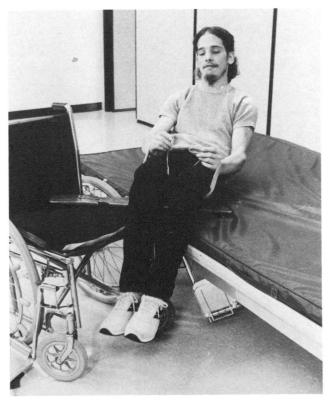

Figure 8–32b

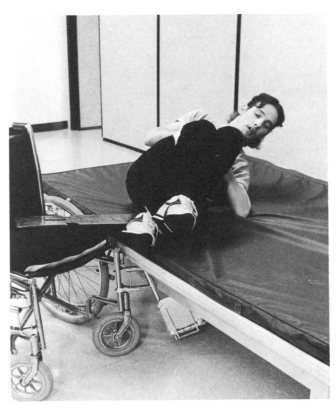

Figure 8–32c

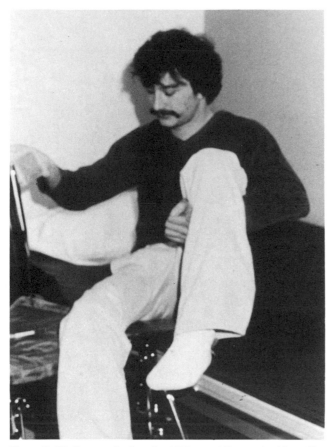

Figure 8–33 One arm is placed on W/C to stabilize trunk while pulling up legs after a transfer.

The patient in Figure 8–33 uses one arm on his W/C to stabilize the trunk while pulling the legs up. This approach still requires good trunk balance as well as good hip flexion.

Some patients choose to put the legs up on the bed before they actually slide out of the W/C (Figure 8–34). The W/C is then used to provide added trunk stability. However, patients with extensor tone may be unable to do this. If they extend their knees, they may initiate a full body extensor pattern and be unable to complete the transfer. Also, remember that even without extensor tone, the slide out of the W/C using this starting position may be more difficult.

Techniques used to move the legs off the bed are often only variations on the themes set getting the legs on the bed. The patient can start from a long sitting position, stabilize with one arm against the W/C, and use his tight finger flexors to lift the leg off the mat or bed (Figure 8–35). Or, he may instead choose to use the mat to stabilize against while he lifts his legs off (Figures 8–36a through 8–36c).

The patient may even decide to slide into the W/C first and then, using the back of the W/C for stability, pull his legs off (Figures 8–37a and 8–37b).

The prone-on-elbows and supine-on-elbows postures can also be modified and used to accomplish this aspect of a transfer.

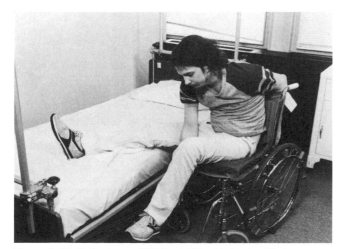

Figure 8–34 Patient uses W/C to stabilize his trunk while he moves his legs onto the bed before his transfer.

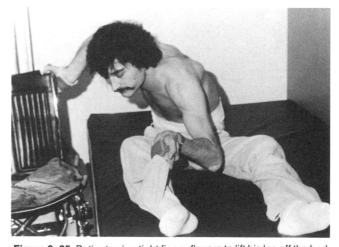

Figure 8–35 Patient using tight finger flexors to lift his leg off the bed.

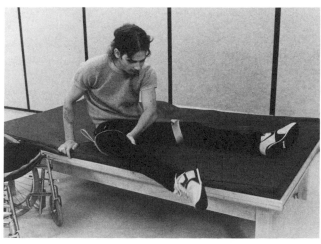

Figure 8–36a Patient uses mat to stabilize against while lifting off his legs.

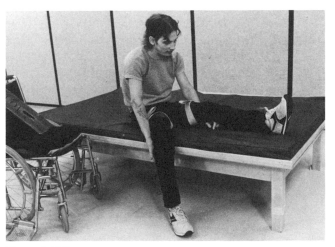

Figure 8–36b

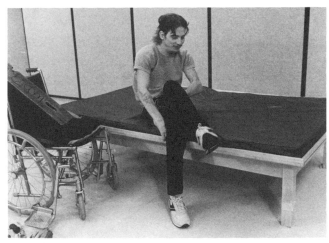

Figure 8–36c Compare position of right arm here to the initial starting position. Because of good sitting balance, the patient is able to narrow his base of support.

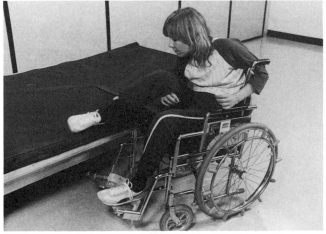

Figure 8–37a Patient lifts legs off the bed using the back of the W/C for stability.

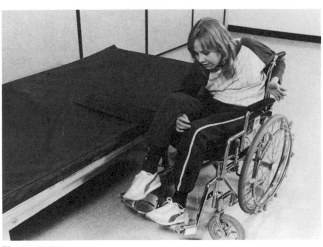

Figure 8–37b

Moving the Buttocks within the W/C

The last thing a patient needs to do after transferring into the W/C is reposition his buttocks back in the chair. Many can accomplish this with a push-up, but there are many who cannot develop enough power to do this.

Most of these patients will have to rely more heavily on body mechanics and incorporate more forward leaning into the process of moving back. This will place much of the body weight forward over the knees, and the buttocks can then be easily levered up and moved back.

The variations in approach are found in hand positions. Some patients are able to put their hands on the rear wheels or their elbows on the armrest, lean forward, and then use scapular depression and shoulder flexors to push the buttocks back. Others lean forward and hook their thumbs inside the armrests. This produces more trunk flexion so less power is needed to push the buttocks back. However, regaining an upright position can be difficult unless the patient has strong pectoralis musculature and a good elbow-locking mechanism.

If the patient has good shoulder extension, he may choose to hook both arms behind his push handles and lean forward. The biceps can then be used to both pull the hips back and regain an upright position.

Dependent Transfers

Each patient needs to have some method of getting in and out of his W/C or bed, even if this will require the maximum assistance of others. As with other types of transfers discussed, many options exist: three-man lifts, two-man lifts, mechanical lifts, or one-man pivots. A patient may be able to provide some minimal assistance with the one-man pivot if he has some scapular depressions and biceps (Figure 8–38). However, no assistance is required of the patient in any of these transfers.

The one-man pivot transfer in Figures 8–39a through 8–39e is done with greater ease than the transfer shown in Figure 8–38. The increased trunk flexion facilitates the move. This transfer also enables the person assisting to keep his back straighter and to use better body mechanics. The patient is able to provide more assistance on the return to the W/C by pushing off the mat.

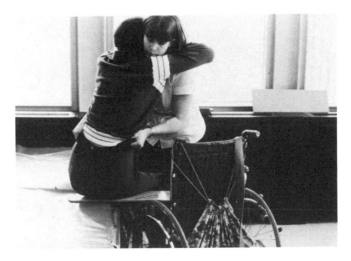

Figure 8–38 One-man pivot transfer. Patient can provide some assistance with the lift by depressing against the therapist's shoulders.

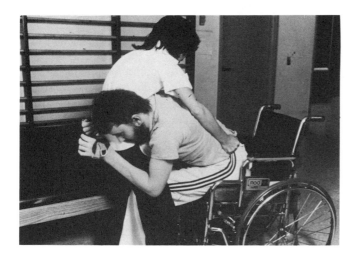

Figure 8–39a One-man pivot transfer.

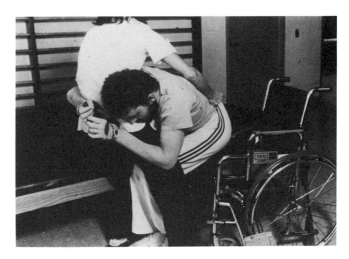

Figure 8–39b

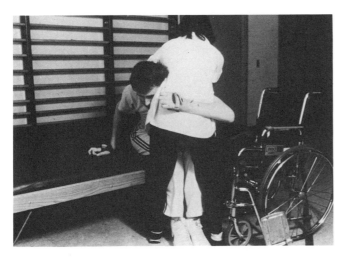

Figure 8–39c

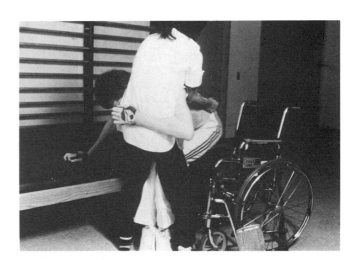

Figure 8–39d

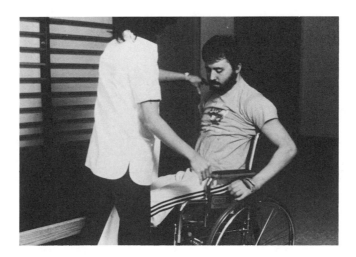

Figure 8–39e

A swivel bar transfer can be useful with the patient who, for whatever reason (e.g., spasticity, ectopic bone, etc.) has limited hip flexion (Figures 8–40a through 8–40d). The trick to this transfer is finding the right height for the swivel bar. It must be low enough for the patient to reach the loop but high enough to allow for the hips to clear the bed. Although the patient needs to supply some assistance with this transfer, hand function is not a necessary requirement; transfers can be accomplished with good shoulder depression and some elbow flexion. Shoulder flexion of at least 140 degrees is essential.

Both the patient doing independent transfers and the patient requiring maximum assistance should be familiar with a transfer that he can use as an alternative in an emergency situation. Dependent transfers can be used in this way. The method chosen will depend very much on patient and family characteristics.

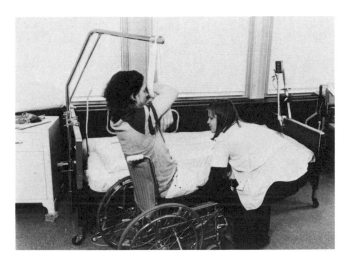

Figure 8–40a A swivel bar transfer.

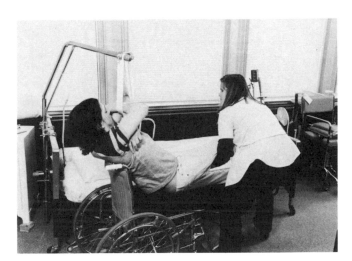

Figure 8–40b

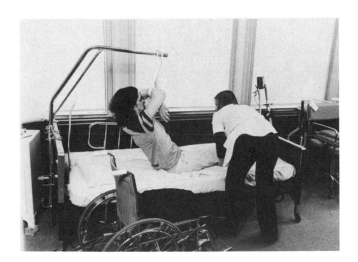

Figure 8–40c

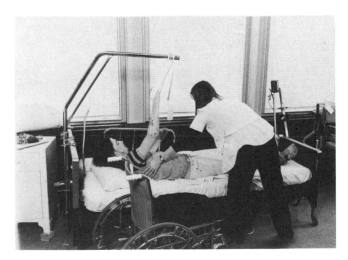

Figure 8–40d

Bathroom Transfers

After the patient has attained a certain degree of proficiency with bed transfers, bathroom transfers are introduced. The techniques of the actual move to and from the W/C and tub or toilet are often much the same as those used by the patient in other transfers. The differences are found in the initial positioning and approach and the equipment being used.

Bathrooms are often small rooms, making positioning difficult, at best. The approaches to bathroom fixtures may need to be more creative, and the patient often has to be satisfied with something less than ideal. The equipment used may feel less stable than the bed. Bath benches and commodes can wiggle. This may mean that slight changes in the angle of push need to be made. While the patient may be able to accomplish a bed transfer using a more horizontal push, he or she may need to incorporate more vertical lines into his push onto a bath bench or commode to prevent it from wiggling and moving away.

Before beginning these transfers, it is important to assess the patient's own bathroom. Both home and work situations should be considered. If a W/C is used, will it fit into the bathroom? Sometimes a W/C narrowing device can facilitate this. Where are the various fixtures positioned in relation to each other? Is there enough room for the W/C to be positioned next to the tub, toilet, or sink? How big is the room? Will there be enough space to turn around? Generally a minimum of five square feet is suggested. The more that is known, the more closely the patient's specific situation can be simulated.

Other considerations should include premorbid preference for hygiene. If the patient prefers a tub bath, why should he be taught skills for the shower? However, present factors are also important. Age, safety, the amount of available assistance, or medical issues may indicate the need for sponge baths. Transfers in and out of the bathroom may take too much time and energy.

If a W/C will fit into the bathroom, the paraplegic can usually transfer directly onto the toilet using some variation of a lateral transfer. Other options may involve approaching the toilet from the front so the patient can pull forward straddling the seat or transferring so that the patient is positioned sideways on the seat.

Approaches will vary depending on the patient and the position of the toilet in the bathroom.

The T8 (sometimes the T6) paraplegic should be able to transfer in and out of the tub bottom. This can be accomplished by transferring first to the edge of the tub. The legs can be moved into the tub either before or after this, depending on the patient. Once positioned at the edge with the legs in the tub, he lowers himself to the bottom. The reverse procedure is used to get out, although this frequently seems to be a little more difficult than getting into the tub.

Probably one of the best situations for the quadriplegic is a roll-in shower. If a commode chair is used, he can transfer directly onto this from the bed. He can roll into the bathroom and over the toilet, do his bowel and bladder care, and then move directly into the shower. Because only one transfer is required, less energy and time are needed.

Some tub benches come with cut-out areas to accommodate bowel and bladder care. The patient is able to transfer from the W/C onto the bench and do both his bowel and bladder care and shower before getting back into the chair. It is often easiest to transfer onto the bench first and then position the legs in the tub. The bench should be far enough back in the tub to allow leg room. Using this equipment, two transfers are required (bed to W/C and W/C to bath bench), but this still requires less energy than separate transfers to the toilet and bath. A shower hose may be used to bring the water closer to the patient and facilitate easier rinsing.

Some patients, however, prefer to transfer directly onto the toilet and into the bath and/or shower. Raised toilet seats, various bath benches, and grab bars should then be considered.

One may also consider devices that automatically regulate water temperature since the quadriplegic is often unable to distinguish between hot and cold. If the patient can be taught to use a part of his body that still has this modality intact, this is preferable.

There is no one way to approach bathroom transfers. As with all transfers, many variations exist. Selection of specific techniques will depend on each individual patient and his specific situation.

It is important to use as little equipment as possible. The more equipment and sophistication needed, the less mobile the patient will be; fewer bathrooms and situations will be accessible to him. If traveling is an issue, the less he has to pack and move around, the better.

Car Transfers

The difficulties with car transfers center around the need to move in such a limited space. Even with the car door opened to its widest position and the front seat positioned as far back as possible, it is still difficult to get a W/C close to the car seat. Longer sliding boards are needed. The car roof is comparatively low. If a mechanical lift is being used, the chains or webbing will have to be shortened to allow for better clearance. Because the space is so small, it is often difficult for someone assisting with a one-man pivot transfer to see. It is not uncommon to have one person designated the sole responsibility of watching the head clearance and helping with positioning during the transfer.

Independent transfers into the car have their own set of special problems. The paraplegic and often the lower quadriplegic patients (C6-C8) can do this. While lateral transfers into the car are fairly easily accomplished, other transfer approaches can be more difficult.

It is hard for example, for the patient to find good hand positions and places to push or pull from. Some patients find that rolling down the window gives them more leverage on the door. (Patients without hand function often do best with electric windows.) Some find that they get better leverage by raising an arm and hooking it on the roof of the car. A locked steering wheel can also provide a stable base to push off of or pull from. Many options exist. Finding the right combination is usually just a matter of experimentation and practice. The legs are usually last into the car and the first out; however, this, too, is open to experimentation.

Some of those able to accomplish independent car transfers are also able to independently bring the W/C into the car. Most paraplegics and sometimes the C8 quadriplegic can do this. After the patient is in the car, he moves the front seat as far forward as possible and removes the foot pedals. He lifts the front casters up onto the floor of the back seat. The patient will need to experiment with various positions and means of stabilizing his trunk. Grasping the front of the chair, he tips it back and pulls it up into the car, rolling the back wheels up and onto the back floor with the casters tipped up over the center hump of the car. The W/C does not necessarily need to go in the back; some prefer to pull the W/C directly into the front passenger side of the car.

There are other options that could be considered: A two-door car will usually provide more space for transferring. Center consoles should be avoided. Power controls for the front seat will position it both forward and backward. Transfers are easier with the seat moved most posteriorly, while the anterior seat position is essential to pulling the W/C into the back seat. A wooden plank could fit onto the floor of the back seat, inclined over the hump. It may facilitate pulling the W/C into the car. No transfer will be required if the patient has a van fitted with a W/C lift and adapted interior to lock the W/C behind the steering wheel.

Wheelchair to Floor Transfers

Getting out of a W/C is fairly easy once the paraplegic patient gets over the initial scare. The patient can scoot to the edge of the chair and come straight out the front or the side of the chair, landing in a hands/knees position (Figures 8–41a through 8–41d) or can straighten out his legs, reach down to the floor and lower himself into a long sitting position (Figures 8–42a through 8–42c).

The latter method or a variation on its theme seems to be the one most frequently preferred. Although it may require a little more strength, it can usually be done with more control than the first method. In addition, the long sitting posture is frequently a more stable position than the hands and knees position.

Frequently, the quadriplegic patient transfers to the floor via a two-man lift or with some mechanical assistance. However, a few are able to transfer independently using a variation of the transfer illustrated in Figures 8–41a through 8–41d.

These patients scoot to the edge of the chair and maintain their head and trunk in extension until the knees have dropped within a few inches of the floor. They may also hook their thumbs into the armrest struts to help control the slide out of the chair. Once they are down as far as possible they will let go of the armrests, flex the head and trunk, and land on the floor either in a prone or a sidelying position on the elbows.

Caution should be exercised in teaching this transfer. Any osteoporotic changes or orthopedic problems would be a contraindication to teaching this transfer. In addition, it would also seem that since most quadriplegics need assistance getting back into the W/C, its usefulness would be limited.

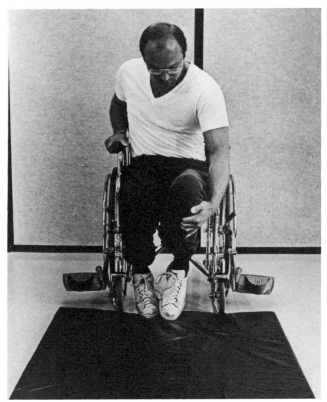

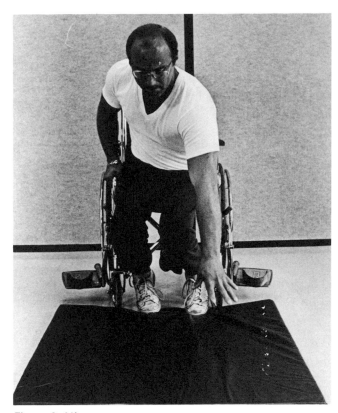

Figure 8–41a Patient is transferring from the W/C to the floor by coming straight out the front and landing in a hands and knees position.

Figure 8–41b

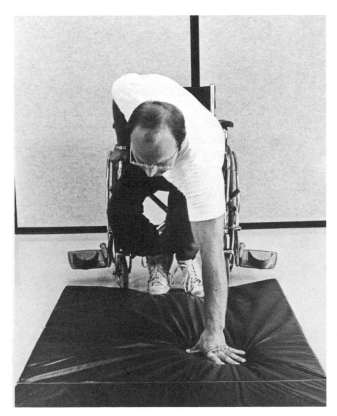

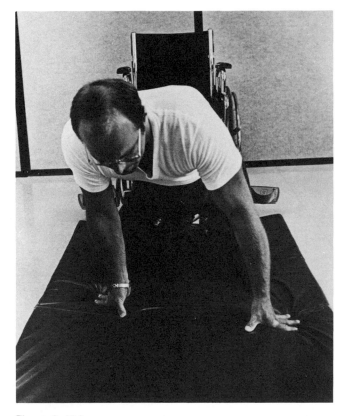

Figure 8–41c

Figure 8–41d

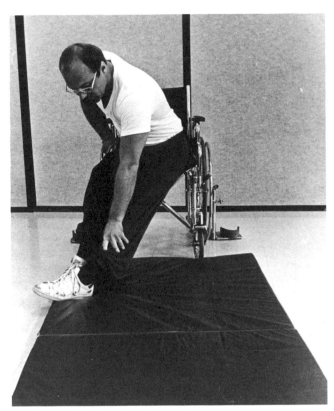

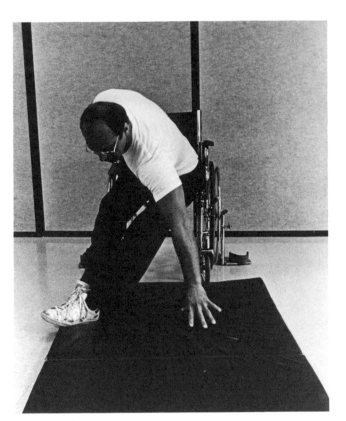

Figure 8–42a Patient straightens his legs, reaches to the floor, and lowers into a long sitting position.

Figure 8–42b

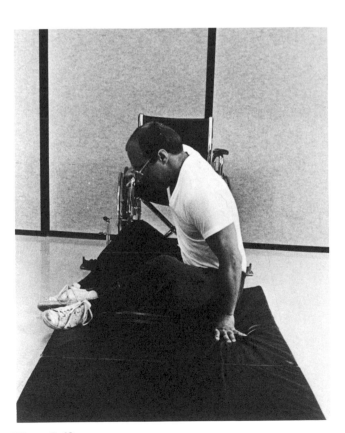

Figure 8–42c

Floor to Wheelchair Transfers

Perhaps the easiest method of moving from the floor into the W/C is to teach the patient first to lift up to an intermediate height, step, or chair and then into the W/C (Figures 8–43a through 8–43e). Although easy and perhaps a good beginning approach, this method is not always practical.

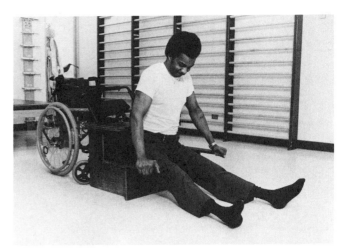

Figure 8–43a Patient lifts up to a step and then into the W/C. To be most successful using this equipment, the patient should place the hands on the step rather than on the step extension, as is shown. The stair might tip if the patient pushes on the extension rather than the step. Once the patient is sitting on the first step, tipping is not a problem.

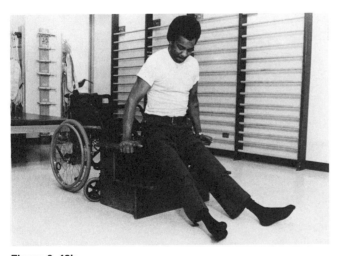

Figure 8–43b

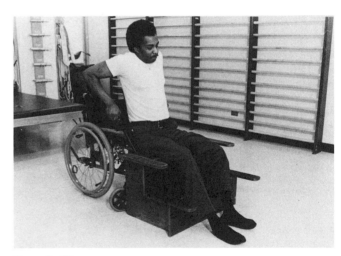

Figure 8–43c

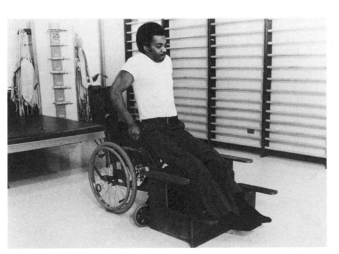

Figure 8–43d

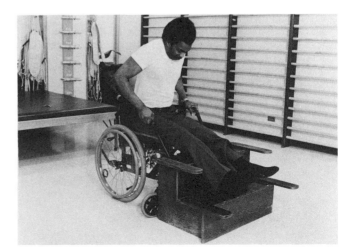

Figure 8–43e

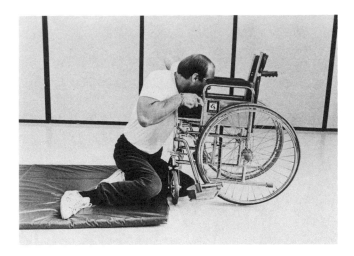

Figure 8–44a Patient uses kneeling position and pulls himself into the W/C.

The patient in Figures 8–44a through 8–44e is illustrating another method. In this approach, the patient must first assume a kneeling position and then pull himself into the W/C. Once in a kneeling posture the transfer is fairly easy. However, getting to kneeling can take a lot of strength and balance. This is another time when short arms can be a real limitation. In order to use this transfer, the patient will need a W/C in which the foot pedals can be moved out of the way.

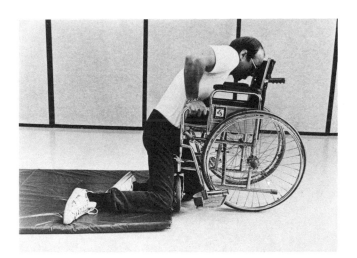

Figure 8–44b

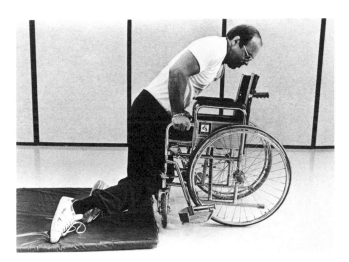

Figure 8–44c

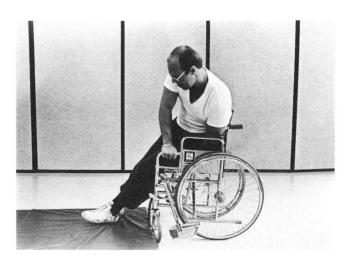

Figure 8–44d

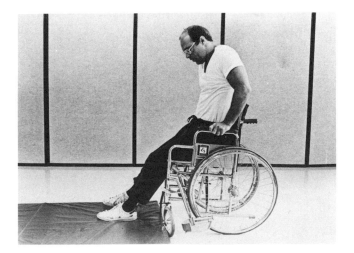

Figure 8–44e

Another method is illustrated in Figures 8–45a through 8–45c. In this case, the starting position is sitting. Notice the leg position. This particular patient is able to set off his extensor tone and use the force of his extending legs to assist in his push back to the W/C.

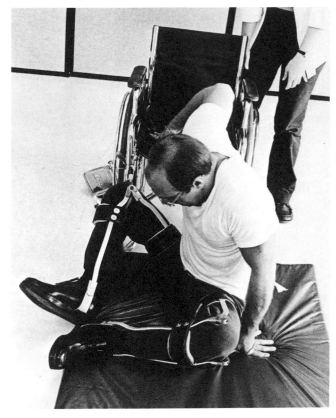

Figure 8–45a Patient transfers from floor to W/C using lower extremity extensor tone to assist the lift.

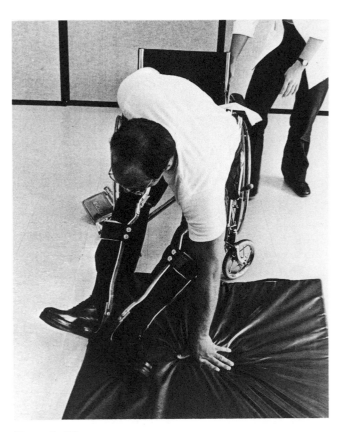

Figure 8–45b

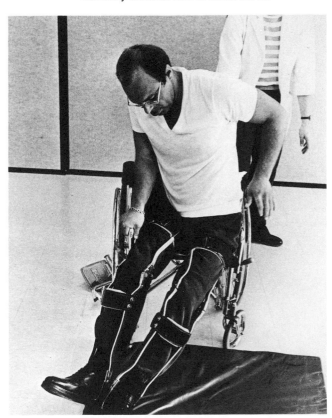

Figure 8–45c

Without the extensor tone to assist, the arms will have to generate more power. The hand position may need to shift to a point where it can give a more vertical push (Figure 8–46). More attention will have to be focused on biomechanics.

Remember to include an element of success in transfer training. One effective way of doing this is initially to decrease the height of the lift. This can be done by stacking floor mats up to the chair or by using portable curbs of varying heights (Figure 8–47). As the patient becomes more proficient with the lift some of the mats can be removed or he can be asked to lift from a smaller curb.

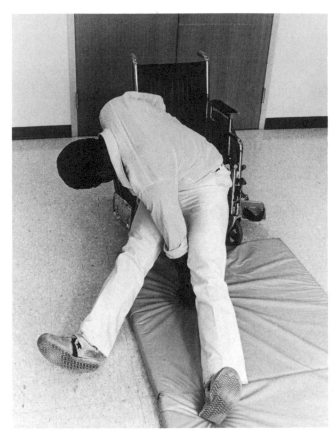

Figure 8–46 Hand position between the legs aids in transfer from floor to W/C. This will place more of the force in a vertical direction, creating more power and ensuring a more successful lift.

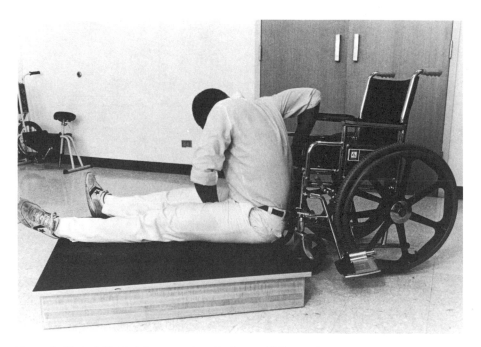

Figure 8–47 An initial training procedure for floor to W/C transfers may include decreasing the height of the lift.

EQUIPMENT OPTIONS

A wide assortment of equipment options exists for the bathroom, including grab bars, raised toilet seats, bath benches, and shower and commode chairs. As with all other equipment decisions, selection is based on the individual patient and his particular needs. Spe-cial emphasis should be placed on safety, ease of trans-fers, stability provided for bathing, and the general mobility provided in the bathroom setting.

A comparison of some bathroom equipment (Ta-ble 8–1), as well as mechanical lifts (Table 8–2), fol-lows.

TABLE 8–1   Comparison of Commode and Shower Chairs*

	E&J	LUMEX	ACTIVE-AIDE (Chairlie)	ACTIVE-AIDE (Craig)
Durability	Will rust, but not as quickly as Active-Aide	Does not rust.	Problems with rust noted by many. (Chairs can be sprayed with special waterproof coating, but many complain that this chips.)	
Comfort	Foot pedals seem to have more adjustability than Active-Aide.		The hard backs of these chairs force the individual to sit straight. Those with balance problems find this uncomfortable.	
	Many seem to find the can-vas back more comfortable.	Many seem to find the can-vas back more comfortable.		
	Floor to seat height is 23 inches.	Floor to seat height is 22 inches.	It may be difficult to accom-modate the tall person because floor to seat height is 19 inches.	Floor to seat height is 23 inches.
	Back height (cushion top-back top) is 14½ inches.	Back height (cushion top-back top) is 18½ inches.	Back height (cushion top-back top) is 12½ inches.	Back height (cushion top-back top) is 16 inches.
	The foam seat is 3 inches thick.	The foam seat is 2 inches thick.	The foam seat is 1 inch thick.	The foam seat is 3 inches thick.
Function	Quad releases are on foot pedals but not on armrests.	Arms drop out of way for transfers but are often diffi-cult to reposition.		A double pan provides more room for hygiene than the Chairlie.
			Armrests can be managed with limited hand function, but footrests cannot.	
	Push handle is standard to facilitate easy mobility for those with balance difficul-ties.	It is 26½ inches wide (with 24 inch wheels), which allows it to fit around toilet tank; however, it may not fit through the bathroom door.	Push handles are available. Push handles are available. Chair measures 25 inches wide with 24 inch wheels, with standard seat width of 17½ inches.	
	It measures 23½ inches wide (with 24-inch wheel).	A regular bed can also be used instead of a bucket.	Chair measures 22 inches wide with four 5 inch casters, with standard seat width of 17½ inches.	
	Foot pedal adjustment is easily maintained—similar to that used in E&J W/C systems.		Chair can be ordered with 15½ inch seat, which will narrow the overall width by 2 inches.	
			Difficult to maintain foot pedal adjustments.	
			Will make custom-size commodes.	
Safety		Because of brake system, some believe that this chair is less stable with the 4 inch caster.		

*All come with option of large rear wheels or four 8 inch casters. Other considerations should include cost and delivery time.

TABLE 8–2   Comparison of Mechanical Lifts

	TRANSAIDE (Lat-2)	HOYER
Patient Comfort	"HD" sling crosses between patient's legs thus allowing patient to feel more secure	Sling cannot be positioned under patient in sitting position; therefore, if patient is transferred to a chair, he has to sit on the sling.
	Sling can be positioned under patient while sitting (this is not done as easily as manufacturer indicates).	Suspension bar is uncomfortable; it does not always seem to be shaped to accommodate heads.
	Four-point suspension cradle seems to accommodate head more comfortably.	
Function	It lifts 300 pounds.	It lifts 400 pounds.
	C-shaped base does not always seem to allow a close approach.	U-shaped base seems to provide more flexibility in how and when it is used.
Assistant Comfort	Base seems a little unsteady.	Hydraulic lift facilitates good body mechanics.
	Hooks occasionally flip out.	
	Crank used to both lift and lower patient.	
	It appears difficult to give patient additional support at the head or to control increases in tone and to manipulate the lift simultaneously using good body mechanics.	

Note: Transaide makes what is called an "institutional lift" that appears functional comparable to the Hoyer (lifts 400 pounds, has U-shaped base) but it is not portable and costs more than the Hoyer.

Transfers—C4 Quadriplegic

Outcome

1. Patient demonstrates ability to direct safe transfers to all surfaces.

Components

a. All aspects of transfer:

- positioning of W/C
- management of W/C parts
- management of equipment used to assist transfer
- actual move from one surface to the next
- supine to sitting and back (including management of lower extremities)

b. Transfer to all surfaces:

- bed
- bath
- toilet
- car
- floor (if indicated)

c. Emergency alternative transfer

Considerations

1. Limitations in ROM, presence of pain, presence of spasticity, and/or pressure sores (could increase difficulty of management and thus make directions more complicated)

2. Respiratory status as it relates to ability to direct care

3. Equipment: What is available to assist?

- mechanical lifts
- bathroom equipment
- hospital bed (with electric bed surface heights easily changed); may make transfer easier

4. Personality prior to injury

- How assertive was patient?

5. Type of transfer (may be determined by characteristics of significant other such as age, medical problems, time demands)

Process

1. Evaluate motor skills.

2. Assess discharge plans and how significant other will be able to assist.

3. Evaluate functional component skills:

- head control
- respiratory skills needed to direct care
- comfort with being handled and moved

4. Improve motor skills.

5. Teach functional component skills.

6. Determine appropriate transfer techniques:

- three-man lifts
- two-man lifts
- one-man lifts
- mechanical lifts

7. Evaluate potential equipment needs (include input from other team members).

8. Teach transfer techniques to patient; include emergency alternative transfer.

9. Determine appropriate equipment.

10. Instruct nursing staff, other team members, and significant others in patient's transfer skills.

11. Incorporate skills into daily routine.

12. Evaluate performance in daily routine.

13. Assist patient in problem solving to alleviate difficulties.

Transfers—C5 Quadriplegic

Outcome

1. Patient demonstrates ability to direct and/or *assist* in safe transfers to all surfaces.

2. Patient demonstrates ability to direct all other transfers.

Components

a. All aspects of transfer:

- positioning of W/C
- management of W/C parts
- management of equipment used to assist transfer
- actual move from one surface to the next
- supine to sitting and back (including management of lower extremities)

b. Transfer to all surfaces:

- bed
- bath
- toilet
- car
- floor

c. Emergency alternative transfer

Considerations

1. *Strength, especially:*

- *scapular depressors*
- *horizontal shoulder adductors*
- *elbow flexors*

2. *ROM: Transfers are easiest if:*

- *shoulder flexion is at least 110 degrees*
- *hip flexion (at least 90 degrees, best if within normal limits)*

3. *Tone*

4. Pain

5. Existing pressure sore or fragile skin (may make directions more difficult)

6. *Body weight, proportions*

7. Equipment: What is available to assist?

- mechanical lifts
- bathroom equipment
- hospital bed (with electric bed surface heights easily changed); may make transfer easier
- *swivel bar*

8. Type of transfer (may be determined by characteristics of significant other, such as age, medical problems, time demands)

Process

1. Evaluate motor skills.

2. Assess discharge plans and how significant other will be able to assist.

3. Evaluate functional component skills:

- head control
- respiratory skills needed to direct care
- comfort with being handled and moved
- *trunk stability on elbows and in sitting*
- *weight-shifting skills on elbows and in sitting*
- *balance and equilibrium reactions on elbows and in sitting*
- *compensatory sensory techniques*
- *skills to compensate for abnormal tone*
- *compensatory movement patterns to accommodate absent musculature*

4. Improve motor skills.

5. Teach functional component skills.

6. Determine appropriate transfer technique:

- three-man lifts
- two-man lifts
- one-man lifts
- mechanical lifts
- *swivel bar*

7. Evaluate potential equipment needs (include input from other team members).

8. Teach transfer techniques to patient; include emergency alternative transfer.

9. Determine appropriate equipment.

10. Instruct nursing staff, other team members, and significant others in patient's transfer skills.

11. Incorporate skills into daily routine.

12. Evaluate performance in daily routine.

13. Assist patient in problem solving to alleviate difficulties.

Transfers—C6 Quadriplegic

Outcome

1. Patient demonstrates ability to assist or *perform* transfers to all surfaces.

2. Patient demonstrates ability to direct transfer to and from floor.

Components

a. All aspects of transfer:

- positioning of W/C
- management of W/C parts
- management of equipment used to assist transfer
- actual move from one surface to the next
- supine to sitting and back (including management of lower extremities)

b. Transfer to all surfaces:

- bed
- bath
- toilet
- car
- floor

c. Emergency alternative transfer

Considerations

1. Strength:

- *shoulders and scapular musculature*
- elbow flexors
- *wrist extensors*

2. ROM: transfers easiest if

- *shoulder flexion and extension within normal limits*
- hips within normal limits

3. Tone

4. *Pain, especially at shoulders*

5. *Coordination*

6. *Endurance (independence can require high endurance levels)*

7. Existing pressure sores or fragile skin (may delay training)

8. Body build, weight, proportions

9. Fear of falling

10. Equipment: What is available to assist?

- *W/C (elevating leg rests hard to manage, get in the way of sliding board)*
- *cushions (some are easier to slide on than others)*
- *sliding boards provide varying amounts of assistance (telescoping sliding boards are easier to position but getting the "slide" of transfer started may be harder; not as much board under patient)*
- *loops*
- *mattresses (firmer mattress usually makes transfer easier)*
- bath and toilet equipment

11. *Age*

Process

1. Evaluate motor skills.

2. Assess discharge plans.

3. Evaluate functional component skills:

- trunk stability on elbows and in sitting
- weight shifting skills on elbows and in sitting
- balance and equilibrium reactions on elbows and in sitting
- compensatory sensory techniques
- skills to compensate for abnormal tone
- compensatory movement patterns to accommodate absent musculature

4. Improve motor skills.

5. Teach functional component skills.

6. Evaluate potential equipment needs (include input from other team members, especially OT and vocational therapist).

7. Teach transfer techniques to patient; include emergency alternative transfer.

8. Determine appropriate equipment.

9. Instruct nursing staff, other team members, and significant others in patient's transfer skills.

10. Incorporate skills into daily routine.

11. Evaluate performance in daily routine.

12. Assist patient in problem solving to alleviate difficulties.

Transfers—C7–8 Quadriplegic

Outcome

1. *Patient demonstrates ability to transfer independently across all level surfaces. (Assistance may be required to get W/C into car.)*

2. *Patient demonstrates ability to assist or independently perform floor transfers.*

Components

a. All aspects of transfer:

- positioning of W/C
- management of W/C parts (brakes, footrests, folding W/C for car transfers)
- management of equipment used to assist transfer
- actual slide from one surface to the next
- supine to sitting and back (including management of lower extremities)

b. Transfer to all surfaces:

- bed
- bath
- toilet
- car
- floor

c. Emergency alternative transfer

Considerations

1. Strength, especially:

- *triceps* (but consider entire upper extremities)

2. ROM, especially:

- hips (at least 90 degrees)

3. Tone

4. Existing pressure sores or fragile skin (may delay training)

5. Age

6. Obesity

7. Equipment: What is available to assist?

- *mechanical lifts to put W/C in car*

Process

1. Evaluate motor skills.

2. Assess discharge plans.

3. Evaluate functional component skills:

- trunk stability in sitting
- weight shifting in sitting
- *ability to lift body weight on extended elbows*
- balance and equilibrium reactions in sitting
- skills to compensate for abnormal tone

4. Improve motor skills.

5. Teach functional component skills.

6. Evaluate potential equipment needs (include input from other team members, especially OT and vocational therapist).

7. Teach transfer techniques (*will probably be a lateral transfer with or without a sliding board*).

8. Determine appropriate equipment.

9. Instruct nursing staff, other team members, and significant others in patient's transfer skills.

10. Incorporate skills into daily routine.

11. Evaluate performance in daily routine.

12. Assist patient in problem solving to alleviate difficulties.

Transfers—Paraplegic

Outcome

1. *Patient demonstrates ability to transfer independently to and from all surfaces both with and without orthosis.*

Components

a. All aspects of transfer:

- positioning of W/C
- management of W/C parts (brakes, footrests, holding W/C for car transfers)
- management of equipment used to assist transfer
- actual slide from one surface to the next
- supine to sitting and back (including management of lower extremities)

b. Transfer to all surfaces:

- bed
- bath
- toilet
- car
- floor

Considerations

1. ROM, especially:

- hips (at least 90 degrees)

2. Tone

3. Obesity

4. Age

5. Existing pressure sores or fragile skin (may delay training)

6. *Orthosis (adds increased width, weight, and bulk to lower extremities)*

Process

1. Evaluate motor skills.

2. Assess discharge plans.

3. Evaluate functional component skills:

- trunk stability in sitting
- weight shifting skills in sitting
- ability to lift body weight on extended elbows
- balance and equilibrium reactions in sitting
- skills to compensate for abnormal tone

4. Improve motor skills.

5. Teach functional component skills.

6. Evaluate potential equipment needs.

7. Teach transfer techniques (will probably be a lateral transfer without a sliding board).

8. Determine appropriate equipment.

9. Instruct nursing staff, other team members, and significant others in patient's transfer skills.

10. Incorporate skills into daily routine.

11. Evaluate performance in daily routine.

12. Assist patient in problem solving to alleviate difficulties.

Wheelchair Mobility

The W/C is a whole new concept for the SCI patient. Prior to his injury he was probably able to walk to get everywhere he wanted to go. Using wheels instead of legs to get around requires a different set of skills. How can these be developed?

ACHIEVING THE OUTCOME

Posture

Achieving good posture should always be one of the first considerations in any attempt to develop W/C skills. Mobility always needs a stable base on which to act. The trunk has to be stable and well aligned before the arms will be free to push the wheels.

Before going further, it should be noted that posture can impact on many other areas of ADL. For instance, it is important for respiration and endurance. The normal curves of the spinal column provide the optimal positioning of the ribs needed for maximal chest expansion. Poor posture can create unequal pressure distribution over the skin, making it more likely for a pressure sore to develop. Good alignment also plays a part in energy conservation. The patient who sits with slumped shoulders and a head positioned forward not only has compromised his respiratory capacity but also has to use more muscle power just to maintain his head position.

Finally good alignment can play a role in prevention of pain. All of us have many asymptomatic idiosyncrasies that can easily become exaggerated with prolonged sitting and cause pain. This is exactly the situation in which the SCI patient finds himself. Most of his waking hours will now be spent sitting.

In general terms, good posture is only a matter of building a stable and symmetrical trunk and head over a level and again stable base of support (pelvis). Symmetry in both the medial-lateral plane and the anterior-posterior plane should be achieved.

Developing this good posture for the SCI patient is not as easy as it might seem. The therapist is always trying to balance stability against mobility. For example, a W/C with a higher back will provide more postural support than one with a lower back. However, if the W/C back is lower, the patient has more freedom and mobility to start his push farther back on the wheel, giving him a longer and faster push.

The patient's skin is another consideration. If trunk supports are used to provide more medial-lateral symmetry, will the patient be able to do independent weight shifts to help prevent the development of pressure sores?

How can good posture be facilitated? For the most part, it can be approached through one of two possible ways—either through proximal points of control or distal points of control.

In that the pelvis is acting as the foundation on which all other symmetry is built, it will be important to start here. The most proximal point of control is the sitting surface. Ideally, a solid non-shifting surface will provide the best support. Pelvic obliquities should not be ignored. Leveling the pelvis can both prevent pressure sores and improve sitting comfort and stability.

Most patients seem to prefer the sling seats of the W/C because of the convenience of easily folding the chair, but this sling seat will also cause lower extremity adduction. This narrows the patient's overall base of support, which may lead to more pelvis and trunk instability. A solid seat or solid seat insert would prevent this. If, however, the patient prefers the sling seat, leg straps might be used instead as a distal point of control holding the legs into some abduction.

The type of cushion used will affect the "shift" of the sitting surface. Gel cushions, for instance, may shift more and not provide as firm a sitting base. In this case the pelvis may again be less stable.

Using distal points of control for the pelvis might include changing the footrest position. However, footrests that are adjusted too high will decrease the support the thighs will be able to provide and thus decrease the overall base of support. Once again the pelvis becomes unstable.

Some raise the footrests in an attempt to prevent the patient from sliding forward out of the seat. A better solution might be found more proximally by slightly inclining the seat to the back (or using a small wedge cushion). This will not only prevent the patient from sliding forward, but may also improve skin pressure distribution by distributing some of the pressure onto the back. To be most effective, this should be done in conjunction with a slightly inclined back support (can be accomplished with a wedge cushion on the back) and a lumbar roll. Without at least the lumbar roll, the pressure over the ischial tuberosities on an inclined seat may be too great. In addition to improved pressure distribution and improved stability, the inclined back may reduce lumbar disc pressure as well as decrease some of the muscle activity in the back muscles.

A lumbar roll is a good distal point of control for the pelvis. This will help maintain the pelvis in a good position as well as prevent kyphosis and minimize scoliosis and pelvic obliquities. It, too, will help balance pressure distribution over the skin by shifting some of the body weight anterior to the ischial tuberosities and over the thighs.

The dimensions of the lumbar roll will vary from patient to patient. Patients with decreased mobility in the lumbar spine may require thinner rolls than those with more mobility in this area. Careful attention should also be taken of shoulder position. If the shoulders are too far back behind the line of gravity, table top activities will be more difficult.

After the pelvis is stable and symmetrical, trunk symmetry and alignment should be evaluated. Frequently nothing further needs to be done, but if this is not the case, a variety of options exist.

Using distal points of control, lap boards, armboards, and adjustable armrests can be provided. These methods can, however, limit functional upper extremity use. More proximal control can be provided by trunk supports.

Remember, posture needs to be looked at not only within the framework of mobility, but of comfort as well. Even if a patient will be mobility dependent, good posture will always lead to improved comfort. So, for instance, adjustable armrests may not be needed to improve trunk symmetry but may be needed to provide more comfort as these will afford one of the few opportunities the SCI patient has to easily change position.

No absolute right and wrong answers exist when trying to determine the best posture for the SCI patient. The compromises made will depend on the patient's physical deficits and his goals.

Advanced W/C Skills in a Manual W/C

Although the presence of some trunk and upper extremity musculature is usually necessary and at the very least makes the performance of advanced W/C skills easier, these skills are primarily a matter of timing and coordination and do not require extreme strength.

Propelling the W/C

The forward push is accomplished through shoulder flexion, adduction, and external rotation. The push backward is accomplished through shoulder extension, adduction, and internal rotation. Trunk flexion and extension movements can be used to add more power to the push.

The patient should avoid putting his thumb on the tire (Figures 9–1a and 9–1b). It will always get caught in the brake. Pull to lock brakes will cut down on some of the thumb bruises, but the thumb should still be on the rim and not on the tire. Only the palm of the hand should be kept on the tire (Figure 9–2).

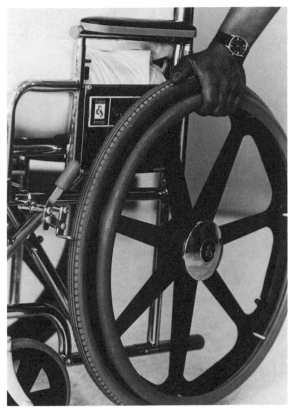

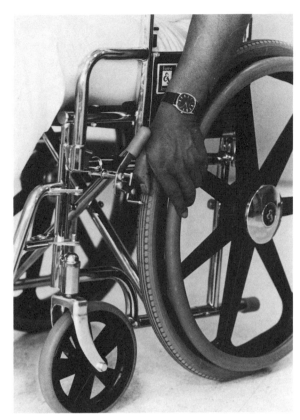

Figure 9–1a Hand is positioned incorrectly. If W/C is pushed in this manner the patient's thumb may get caught on the brake.

Figure 9–1b

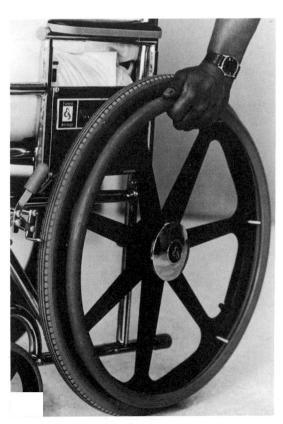

Figure 9–2 Hand is positioned correctly with thumb on rim of wheel.

Wheelies

The wheelie is perhaps the cornerstone of all advanced W/C skills. Initially the patient is placed in the wheelie and asked to maintain it. Spotting with at least one hand on the patient's shoulder will give him a better sense of how he is actually doing. If both hands are kept under the push handles of the W/C, the patient has no idea whether he is maintaining the position or being held in it by the spotter.

After he has acquired some sense of where this position is and feels comfortable with it, he then learns how to assume the position. This is usually taught in three steps. Keeping his hands on the wheels, the patient wheels (1) forward, (2) backward, and (3) then forward again as he leans back in the chair and pops up to a wheelie. The patient can work on this independently using a setup such as the one shown in Figure 9–3. Although triceps are usually needed, timing and coordination seem more important than strength. The rhythm of moving the wheel forward, back, and then forward again frequently makes the activity easier; however, many patients drop the first two steps as they acquire more skill. If done with skill, the head and shoulders should be relaxed.

When the patient has learned to assume and maintain a wheelie, he must learn to move forward, to move back, and to turn in the wheelie position. This is usually only a matter of practice.

Rough terrain, including gravel and mud, is probably best negotiated in a wheelie position. Even if a patient is unable to do a wheelie he should be able to instruct others in how to push the W/C in this position.

Falling in the W/C

All independent W/C users should be familiar with what to do if they fall while in the W/C. A patient only needs to remember to tuck his head and use an arm to block his knees, preventing them from hitting his face. If this is done, the patient will slide out the back of his W/C unharmed. When able, most patients prefer to use one arm to hold onto the W/C. This will keep the buttocks in the W/C and prevent the slide out the back (Figures 9–4a through 9–4c).

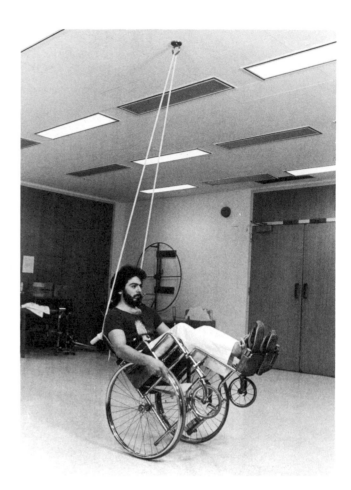

Figure 9–3 This setup is one method that can be used to teach a wheelie.

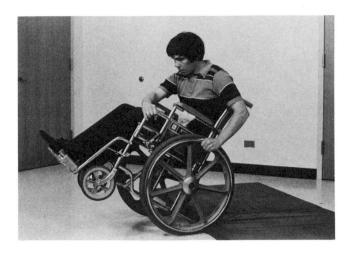

Figure 9–4a Falling in the W/C

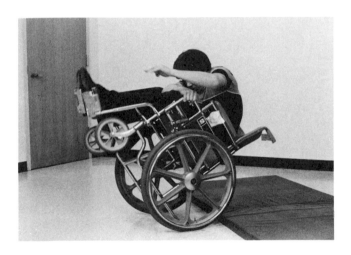

Figure 9–4b

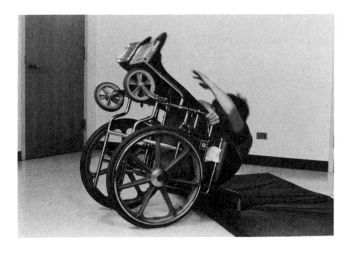

Figure 9–4c

Regaining an Upright Position in the W/C after a Fall

With a little practice, the patient should be able to regain an upright position without getting out of the W/C (Figures 9–5a through 9–5f). He remains sitting in the W/C with his feet hanging off the foot pedals; the brakes are locked. With one arm behind the W/C and the other crossing the midline and pushing on the front of the W/C, the patient pushes with the back hand and "walks" the chair up to an upright position. The stronger, more coordinated patient will be able to do this with the back arm inside the push handle. The task can be made easier, however, if the back arm is placed outside the push handle. This will facilitate more trunk flexion.

If the above method is too difficult, the patient always has the option of getting out of the W/C, tipping it back to the upright position, and then doing a transfer into the chair from the floor.

Ramps

Very few special techniques are required to maneuver on a 1:10 ramp; the steeper ramps, however, require a little more skill. To ascend, the patient should jump the wheels on the ramp, lean forward into the ramp, and push. Leaning forward is required to prevent a backward tip. Ramp retarders may facilitate the climb. However, most patients learn to let go of the wheel while they still have some forward momentum and so have time to catch the wheel in a new position before they start to roll backwards. If the ramp is long but wide, the person may consider ascending diagonally or in a zigzag manner.

Descending a steep ramp backward is perhaps the easiest and safest method. Again, the patient needs to lean forward into the ramp to prevent tipping. Quicker options for descent would include descending forward in a diagonal zigzag manner or forward in a wheelie position—usually the more preferred method.

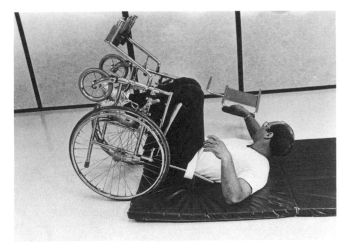

Figure 9–5a Patient is attempting to regain an upright position after a fall. The front hand pushes on the front of the W/C, and the back hand is used to push up from the floor.

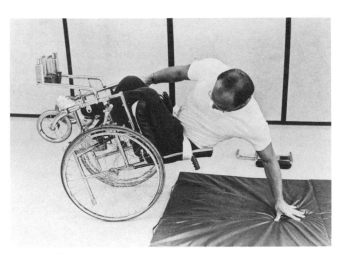

Figure 9–5b

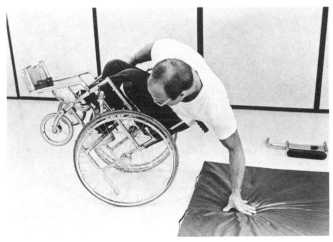

Figure 9–5c At this point, if strength is limited rocking the W/C forward can help.

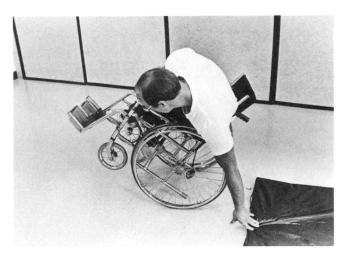

Figure 9–5d Note head position and trunk flexion.

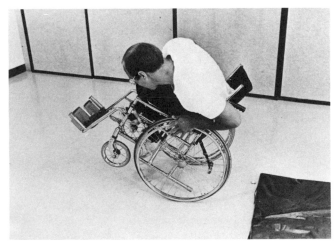

Figure 9–5e

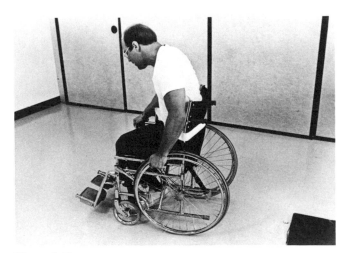

Figure 9–5f

Curbs—Up

A patient can usually maneuver up a 2-inch curb without using a full "wheelie." He should approach the curb, stop, pop the front casters up onto the curb, lean forward, and push the rear wheels up. After he has acquired a little skill, he probably will be able to do the maneuver without first stopping at the curb to pop up the front casters.

Higher curbs require a longer approach (5-10 feet) to build up momentum. The patient should approach the curb in a wheelie, drop the front casters onto the curb, lean forward, and then push up the rear wheels. Rhythm and timing are needed to be successful. The patient may want to wait to pop the wheelie until just before he gets to the curb; however, this usually requires more timing. Many find it more difficult to assume a wheelie "on the move."

Curbs—Down

One of the easiest ways to descend a curb is backward. The patient backs to the edge of the curb and stops. Holding the rear wheels, he leans forward and slowly lowers the W/C down. He should make sure that the wheels come off the curb evenly, otherwise the chair is likely to tip. Once the back wheels are down, he should pivot the front casters off.

Although a little more difficult, most patients prefer descending a curb forward using a wheelie. It is quicker. Once off the curb, however, the patient should drop the casters quickly so that the chair does not tip backward.

Intermediate W/C Skills in a Manual W/C

The SCI patient with a higher level of injury often has difficulty with just the rhythmic pushing of a manual W/C. This is easily understood when one considers the decreases in sensation and shoulder pain that are often found along with the strength deficits. In addition, immobilization devices of the head and trunk restrict movement, making it hard to see.

Various accessories can be added to the W/C to facilitate W/C mobility. Projections can be attached to the wheel rim. Oblique projections are easier to push than the vertical, but these add width to the chair. Some complain that the projections get caught in shag rugs and grass and so prefer to use the plastic-coated W/C rims with leather mitts. Projections also seem to encour-

age more of a "biceps" push. This can lead to a biceps and/or supination contracture, which may in turn interfere with feeding and table-top activities, among other things. Using the plastic-coated rims or catheter tubing around the rim encourages the patient to push with more elbow extension and use more pronation. Many also believe that it is easier to get into the rhythm of pushing when they use the plastic-coated rims (as opposed to the projections). However, this kind of rim may not provide the patient with enough grip to perform some of the higher level skills.

Obviously, the lighter the W/C, the easier it is to push. Pneumatic tires are often easier to push outside but can be more difficult indoors on carpets.

It is easier to propel the W/C forward than backward. The latter is frequently only accomplished by maximum shoulder depression and exaggerated head and neck extension.

Turns can be done in the usual way by simultaneously pushing forward on one wheel and back on the other. Brake extensions may also be used to facilitate this. If the patient wants to turn to the right, he locks the right wheel and pushes with the left hand. The reverse procedure is used to turn to the left. This second technique requires less energy, but the turn is not as sharp.

It is important that the patient be comfortable with as many different terrains as possible. Increased strength and body momentum are required as the terrain becomes more difficult. If rough ground is not available, this can be simulated by having the patient push over floor mats.

Even though independence on curbs and ramps may be an unrealistic goal for many patients with higher level injuries, it is still important that these subjects be introduced. Knowledge of some of these techniques may help them handle all the cracks and bumps in sidewalks, making them more independent on level surfaces. They may be able to use their brakes to help control the buildup of speed as they descend ramps. At the very least, they should be able to instruct others to assist with these activities (even if they will primarily be using an electric W/C).

Advanced W/C Skills in an Electric W/C

Advanced W/C skills also exist for the electric W/C user. Many of these skills are based not only on the patient himself but also on a good understanding of the particular electric W/C being used and the controls selected to operate it.

For example, many electric W/Cs will automatically reduce speed with turns. Using this information, a patient may be able to gain more control going down a ramp by descending in a series of short turns. A sharper turn can be accomplished in many of these W/Cs if initiated from a dead stop rather than from a forward movement. This is because when turning from a stationary position, both motors of the W/C will engage, one forward and the other backward. A turn initiated from an already moving W/C is done with only one motor.

Each patient should be intimately aware of how his electric W/C works. Owners' manuals are provided with all W/Cs. With a good working knowledge of how his W/C performs, the electric W/C user will be able to move with skill and ease.

EQUIPMENT OPTIONS

A W/C is not just something an individual uses to get from one place to the next. For the disabled, it becomes an integral part of his self-image and in many ways will help define his life style.

The goal in selecting a W/C is to find the lightest and the narrowest one possible that will still meet the individual patient's special needs. This will help eliminate, or at least minimize, accessibility issues.

W/C weight is often a compromise between durability and function. Added accessories should be kept to a minimum, since they will always increase the weight of the W/C.

When looking at the W/C width, consider both seat width and the back width. Seat width should include enough space to fit one's hands on either side of the patient's hips. The W/C back uprights should frame the patient's back, not compromise it. In addition to the basic frame construction, wraparound armrests might also be considered to narrow the chair. Pneumatic tires add more width to the chair than solid tires, and oblique projections can add one and one-half to two inches to W/C width, depending on how oblique the projections are. Narrowing devices can also be considered to decrease overall width.

For more specifics on W/C prescription refer to the equipment guidelines at the beginning of this manual and to the section on posture at the beginning of this Unit as well as the many standard sources for W/C fit. Compromises will always have to be made between weight and function, comfort and accessibility, stability and mobility, and so on. But one can make a good decision only after exploring all the options.

Other considerations are included in Tables 9–1 through 9–3. Please note that all comparisons are made in reference to top-of-the-line W/Cs.

SPECIAL PROBLEMS

Obese Individuals

The obese patient in need of a custom-size W/C presents some unusual problems. For every two inches of extra width in an adult size E&J chair, the seat height raises one inch. This creates problems for sitting at a table or for lateral transfers. On request, for an additional fee, the manufacturer can reduce the crossbar length to correct this. The seat height is not automatically raised in the oversized W/C made by other manufacturers.

The frame may have to be welded on the E&J W/C for the patient who weighs over 350 pounds. Transporting such a W/C is a problem if it does not fold. Also, extra wide W/Cs may not fit on the standard ramps of vans used for public transportation.

E&J will not make an electric W/C for the patient weighing over 350 pounds. Rolls, however, does not seem to have a weight limit.

Hip Disarticulation

Paraplegics who have had bilateral hip disarticulations but who are not in a prosthesis or wear it inconsistently present another W/C problem. A reclining W/C, with cushions for seat and back, is a possibility. The patient may be encouraged to lie prone and propel the wheels like a cart. When the patient is in the prosthesis, a solid seat insert can be used and the back raised for standard W/C propulsion.

TABLE 9–1   Comparison of Manual Wheelchairs

Function	E & J	Rolls	Quadra	Stainless	Quickie
Management of Wheelchair Parts	Accessories to facilitate easy management are available, but generally cost more. (Not all accessories are available in lower priced models.)	Accessories such as quad releases for armrests and foot pedals come standard on all wheelchairs in the 900 and 700 series. (Not always available in other series.)	Armrests: Often hard to get on and off initially, takes awhile to "wear in." Swing-away armrests: May be more difficult for quads to manage (but can be done with practice.) Armrests that lift up and out are also available.	Quad releases for armrests and foot pedals are available at an extra charge. Quad lever release on armrests can be mounted either on the inside or outside of the arm frame. Foot pedals will lift off from the front of the W/C. (Other W/Cs require that the pedals be swung to the side before lifting off.) Pedals will stand on their own, so it is easier for a person to reach and reattach to W/C.	Swing-away footrests are not available. Caster pin locks can more easily be managed by those with quadriplegia. Most accessories (including such things as push handles, brakes) are available, but at an extra charge.
			Quick release wheels are standard.	Quick release wheels available at an extra charge.	Quick release wheels (both front and back) are a standard option.
Transfers	Armrests are ½ inch higher than Rolls.	Armrests seem to be ½ inch lower than E&J; wheelchair to floor transfers may be more difficult.	Because chair is so light, wheelchair stabilization is more difficult. Quadriplegics who need more stabilization may be unable to transfer to and from this wheelchair.		Wheelchair stabilization during transfers may be difficult for quadriplegics because wheelchair is lighter.
Wheelchair Propulsion	Sealed precision bearing wheels available as standard option on all premier W/Cs.	Sealed precision bearing wheels available in 900, 700, and 500 series.	May be easier to push because it is lighter than many standard adult W/Cs. Sealed precision bearing wheels are a standard option.	Precision bearing wheels available at no extra charge.	Lighter wheelchair, so may be easier to push than many standard adult W/Cs. Sealed precision bearing wheels are a standard option. A low mount brake option is available that will facilitate a longer push.
Assumption of Standing			Assumption of standing may be more difficult due to problems with wheelchair stabilization.		Assumption of standing may be more difficult due to problems with wheelchair stabilization.

TABLE 9–1   continued

Function	E & J	Rolls	Quadra	Stainless	Quickie
Use of BFO		Upholstery may need to be remounted to accommodate BFO	BFOs are hard to use with this chair. Lapboard is difficult to accommodate.		BFOs are hard to use with this chair. Lapboard is difficult to accommodate.

Comfort

	E & J	Rolls	Quadra	Stainless	Quickie
	Choice of modular back heights a standard option only on light weight Premier and stainless models. (12½; 14½; 16½; 18½; 20½)	Choice of back heights available in 700, 500 and 900 series. (11½; 14½; 15½ . . .)	Choice of back height is standard option. (7-11 inches; 11-15 inches; 15-19 inches)	Choice of modular back height is a standard option. (12 inches; 14 inches; 16 inches; 18 inches; 20 inches)	Choice of back height is a standard option. (8½-12 inches; 12-15½ inches; 15-19 inches)
			Quadriplegic patients often do not feel well-supported (feel like they will fall out of wheelchair).	Fit of wheelchair parts is tighter, so chair does not rattle as much as others might.	Foot pedals can be mounted behind or in front of the extension tubing as well as inclined.
			Fixed footrests do not seem flexible enough to provide foot position patients desire. The removable footrests are somewhat better.		Front riggings for footrests are available in 3 lengths (short, medium, and long) and are adjustable within 3 inches.
			Trunk supports are difficult to attach.		Trunk supports may be difficult to attach.
	Tall chairs are available as a standard option only in the light weight Premier (seat depth 17 inches; back height 18½ inches; seat height is not raised).	Tall chairs are available as standard option in 700 and 900 series (back height seat depth and height are all raised 2 inches).		Tall chairs are available as a standard option (seat height 22 inches; seat depth 17 inches; back height 18 inches).	Standard seat depth is 15 inches but patient can get seat depths from 12 inches - 17 inches with an additional charge.
	Low seat (17½ inches from floor) is available as a standard option.	Low seat (17 inches from floor) available as standard option.		Low seat (17½ inches from floor) is available as a standard option (uses 20 inch wheel).	Armrests can be bolted on at different heights (within 3 inches).

TABLE 9–1   continued

Accessibility	E & J	Rolls	Quadra	Stainless	Quickie
Turning Radius	Generally needs at least 5 square feet in which to turn.	Foot pedals are contoured at corners to decrease turning radius (seems to decrease radius by at least 1 inch). 500 series—caster position can be changed to increase or decrease turning radius. Symmetrical repositioning of casters seems easier than Quadra.	Caster position can be changed to increase or decrease turning radius as desired; however, it may be difficult to set both casters at exactly the same point.	Generally needs at least 5 square feet in which to turn.	Generally needs at least 5 square feet in which to turn.
Weight (as stated by the various companies)*	Standard weight is 45 lbs. (without front riggings). Active duty LW is 35-37 lbs. Quicksilver (stainless) is 38 lbs. (without front riggings).	Standard weight is 45-46 lbs. HPL is 37-38 lbs. Rollite is 29 lbs. 700 Series (stainless) is 37 lbs. 500 Series (Titanium) is 27 lbs.	Adult folder, fully rigged, weighs 25 lbs.	Catalina Rx-30 (top-of-the-line W/C) weighs 37 lbs. (with the front riggings).	With wheels it weighs approximately 24 lbs.; without wheels it weighs 12 lbs.
Width	A 14 inch seat wheelchair is available, but not in the Premier line. 15; 16; 17; and 18 inch seats are available in the Premier line. A custom order is required for seat widths greater than 18 inches. Seat height will be raised 1 inch for every 2 inch increase in width unless otherwise specified. There is a weight limitation on folding oversized W/Cs.	Slim model (14 inch seat width) is available in top-of-the-line series. Seat widths of both 20 inch and 22 inch are available in top-of-the-line series. Seat widths greater than 22 inches require a custom order. Seat height will not be raised as width is increased. There does not seem to be a weight limitation.	A custom order is required for seat widths greater than 18 inches and less than 16 inches.	11 inch-20 inch seat widths are a standard option. Will make folding oversized W/C. There is no weight limitation.	12 inch-20 inch seat widths are available (company will go wider but not smaller).

*Weight is often a difficult thing to assess because of the accessories that may or may not be included in the base weight. There seems to be no standard between companies.

TABLE 9–1   continued

Durability	E & J	Rolls	Quadra	Stainless	Quickie
	Quicksilver (stainless model) side frame and x-bars have a lifetime guarantee. Mag wheels are not painted so they may be more durable.	Mag wheels are painted. This can chip. Some patients complain of cuts from the paint chips.	Urethane wheels are available. The frame has lifetime guarantee. However, the frame does seem to get "bent-up" easily. The frame is rust free. New modifications are made to accommodate older model wheelchairs, so a new wheelchair does not have to be purchased. Some patients feel that the upholstery tears and stretches more easily than both Rolls and E & J.	The entire wheelchair is stainless. (Both E & J and Rolls have accessory parts on their stainless chairs that are not stainless.) It is rust-proof and can be steam cleaned. There is a life warranty on side frames and cross braces. Replacement parts for Catalina Rx-30 series are standardized. Heliarc weld is used, so if chair frame does crack, any welder can fix this; the wheelchair does not have to go back to the company. Urethane tires are available. Tips on brakes and projections are urethane instead of rubber, which tears and rips more easily.	Has a telescoping folding mechanism (rather than a floating seat). The company claims this will be more durable. Aircraft aluminum is used to make the frame. It has adjustable sliding axle mounts (rather than holes). The company claims this system will better absorb shock and decrease the possibility of bending an axle. Projections on the hand rim are individually bolted on, so if you break one, you don't have to replace the whole rim. Urethane casters are a standard option. Gortex upholstery is durable, light, breathes, and is moisture resistant.
Cosmesis*	There is a wide variety of upholstery colors in the Premier line. Quicksilver is only available in Silvergray. The company recently added the Lightning W/C to its Premier line. This chair does not have the traditional "wheelchair look."	In the 900 series, upholstery attaches differently than in E & J; it gives a slightly different look. It has hook push handles and padded side arm panels. There are limited upholstery color options. The 500 series offers a style with a less traditional "wheelchair look."	The frame is available in 10 different colors, but many feel that the chair does not have the traditional "wheelchair look." The upholstery color options are limited.	There is a wide variety of upholstery colors. As with all stainless chairs, this wheelchair does not have the shiny chrome finish.	The frame is available in twelve different colors. Upholstery color options are limited to black. It does not have the traditional "wheelchair look."

*Most companies now offer at least one sport style (or less traditionally styled) W/C; but a more comprehensive comparison of comparable styles is beyond the scope of this manual. For a more specific comparison of the sport W/Cs, refer to the *Sports 'N Spokes* magazine. It annually does a comparison of these chairs.

TABLE 9–2   Comparison of Standard Electric Wheelchairs*

	E & J	Rolls
Durability	Heavy-duty caster forks and construction are available, but require an additional charge. However, chairs come standard with spring-loaded casters, which E&J states provide better shock absorption. So heavy duty forks should not be needed.	The chair automatically comes with heavy-duty caster forks and gussetted frame.
Management of Wheelchair Parts	It is difficult to engage the motor.	The motor is easier to engage.
	The batteries are removable, but with difficulty.	The batteries seem to be more easily removed.
Propulsion	Gets 11 miles/charge.	
	Two control options are available: • proportional speed—up to 5.0 mph on proportional. When on "low" will go up to 3.6 mph. • preset 4-speed—¾ to 3 mph.	Control options: Only proportional control is available (5 mph). Some find this speed too fast. Servicemen can adjust this to a lower setting (this is not possible with E&J).
	Features an acceleration limiting function that E&J states provides for smoother starts.	Regenerative braking (speed is more controlled going down ramps). Because of this, W/C can get 22 miles/charge.
	There is a two-stage braking system that E&J states provides for smoother stops.	Directional control—W/C will go straight, even on a slanted sidewalk without a correction by user.

*Most of the comments regarding manual W/Cs can be applied to electric W/Cs. These are some additional considerations.

TABLE 9–3   Wheelchair Accessories

	Advantages	Disadvantages
Armrests		
Adjustable height	Facilitate more comfortable arm position	Tend to rattle
	Can be raised to facilitate standing and W/C to floor transfers	
	Can be lowered 1 inch more than standard armrest	
Wrap-around armrests	Reduce width of W/C by at least 1 inch	Arms cannot be turned around to assist patients to stand
		May be more difficult for the quadriplegic to manage
Trough armrests	Can facilitate more comfortable arm positioning	Can add as much as 3 inches to the overall W/C width (this can be set in 1 inch if needed)
Retractable trough armrests	Can be used on either standard or electric reclining W/C	See "trough armrests"
Footrests		
Swing-away	Usually preferred over elevating legrests because of lighter weight and manageability	
Elevating legrests	May help decrease orthostatic hypertension and lower extremity edema	Lateral transfers are more difficult because of position on W/C
	Usually come with large foot plate	Heavier than swing-away footrests
	May be easier to accommodate individuals with long legs	May increase turning radius of W/C
Wheels		
Solid tires	Most easily maintained; do not go flat	Not considered to give the smoothest ride
	Add less width to W/C than pneumatic	Not recommended for curb jumping
Pneumatic tires (1¼ inches, essentially a 24-inch bicycle tire)	Smoother ride	Go flat
	Can be used to jump curbs	May be harder to push, especially on carpets
Precision-bearing	Requires less maintenance than other wheels	More expensive than other wheels
	Different bearing system seems to require less effort to push	
	May be used as a compromise by the patient who would need the lighter W/C for easy propulsion but needs more support than many of the sport-style W/Cs seem able to offer	
Mag wheel	It is a stronger wheel	It is 1½ lbs heavier than pneumatics
	It is a more durable wheel	
Casters		
Solid casters	More easily maintained	Not considered to give the smoothest ride
	Only add 2¾ pounds to W/C	Wheels tend to get caught easily; hard to push over gravel
Semipneumatic	Puncture proof	Add approximately 5½ pounds to W/C
	Easier to push over sidewalks, elevator cracks, gravel	Propulsion over carpeting may be more difficult

TABLE 9–3   continued

	Advantages	Disadvantages
Pneumatic	Possibly provide a smoother ride	Another tire to go flat
Urethane (Some companies also have 24-inch urethane tires)	• Less maintenance than pneumatics but still seems to provide smooth ride • Compromise between solid tire and pneumatic tire. Gives a smoother ride than solid tires but not as smooth as pneumatic tires • Easier to propel on solid ground than solid tires because wheel surface comes to a point	Vendors may have more difficulty replacing these tires
Back Inserts	Provides more stability May be used to add extra back support on a temporary basis	Depending on type used, may decrease seat depth Not as much mobility with higher backs (lower backs facilitate a faster push) If not attached to W/C, will tend to fall through between seat and back upholstery
Ramp Retarders	Prevents rolling back on an incline so may be easier to push up hills/ramps (allows forward movement only, letting hands move forward to propel or open doors)	Add approximately 2 pounds to weight of W/C
Caster Pin Locks	Prevents W/C from moving during transfers	Add approximately 1 pound to weight of W/C
Trunk Positioners		
MED trunk supports	Inexpensive	May interfere with independent lateral transfers Cannot be used with electric reclining W/C systems because of sheering forces during reclining
E&J trunk positioners	Many possible adjustments and positions Can be maintained on armrests, leaving space on W/C side frame for BFO mounts, and so on	Unless permanently glued, positions frequently difficult to maintain Tend to break with excessive pressure Expensive
Spherical thoracic supports	Can be swung out of the way for transfers	Can only be attached to back side frames. On quad systems W/C, often no room to mount
Rolls trunk supports	Inexpensive Seems to provide and maintain many adjustment options	Can only be attached to back side frames Upholstery screws have to be removed to slide attaching ring mount into place
Narrowing Devices	Allows up to 4 inch reduction in overall W/C width	Adds approximately 1½ pounds to weight of W/C May be difficult to operate
Quad Footrest Releases for Cam Locks	Facilitates swinging away footrests	More difficult to get back on W/C once off Adds weight to W/C
Heavy-duty Caster Forks	Increases durability of W/C Should be especially considered for the active curb jumper or the very heavy patient	Adds weight to W/C

Wheelchair Mobility—C4 Quadriplegic

Outcome

1. Patient demonstrates ability to maneuver motorized W/C independently on all smooth level surfaces. Assistance may be required on elevations and rough ground (patient will usually not be able to use upper extremities for controls).

2. Patient demonstrates ability to direct when assistance is required.

Components

a. Both manual and electric W/C

b. Forward-backward turns

c. Management of all W/C parts (brakes, legrests)

d. Management of doors

e. Indoors:

- all surfaces, tile to carpet
- doorways
- maneuvering in tight places
- elevators
- elevations

f. Outdoors:

- all terrains
- elevations (ramps, curbs, bumps, and cracks in sidewalk)
- crossing streets safely

Considerations

1. Strength:

- neck musculature
- what movement patterns are available?

2. Respiratory status (as it relates to ability to direct care)

3. Equipment: What is available to assist?

- type of W/C
- type of controls

4. Personality prior to injury

- How assertive was patient?

Process

1. Evaluate motor skills.

2. Assess potential architectural barriers.

3. Evaluate functional component skills:

- head control
- respiratory skills needed to direct care
- manipulation of W/C controls

4. Improve motor skills.

5. Teach functional component skills.

6. Evaluate type of W/C and controls needed (consider consulting OT and research and engineering, if available).

7. Create trunk stability in W/C.

8. Teach W/C skills. When using electric W/C, consider teaching basic operation of controls in simulator or with W/C motor disengaged.

9. Increase endurance with W/C skills.

10. Determine appropriate W/Cs.

11. Instruct nursing staff, other team members, and significant other in patient's W/C mobility skills.

12. Incorporate skills into daily routine.

13. Evaluate performance in daily routine.

14. Assist patient in problem solving to alleviate difficulties.

Electric Wheelchair Mobility—C5 Quadriplegic

Outcome

1. Patient demonstrates ability to maneuver motorized W/C *(using hand controls)* independently on all smooth level surfaces. Assistance may be required on elevations and rough surfaces.

2. Patient demonstrates ability to direct when assistance is required.

Components

a. Forward-backward turns

b. Management of all W/C parts (brakes, ramp retarders)

c. Management of doors

d. Indoors:
   - all surfaces, tile to carpet
   - doorways
   - maneuvering in tight places
   - elevators
   - elevations

e. Outdoors:
   - all terrains
   - elevations (ramps, curbs, bumps, and cracks in sidewalk)
   - crossing streets safely

Considerations

1. Strength, *especially serratus anterior, scapular adductors, but also:*
   - *shoulder flexors*
   - *elbow flexors*

2. ROM: at least 90 degrees for hips to fit into standard adult W/C

3. Tone: *Particularly increase in upper extremities (may interfere)*

4. Respiratory status (as it relates to ability to direct care)

5. Equipment: What is available to assist?
   - type of W/C
   - type of controls

6. Personality prior to injury
   - How assertive was patient?

Process

1. Evaluate motor skills.

2. Assess potential architectural barriers.

3. Evaluate functional component skills:
   - head control
   - *trunk stability in sitting*
   - *balance and equilibrium reactions in sitting*
   - *use of upper extremities in sitting*
   - respiratory skills needed to direct care
   - manipulation of W/C controls

4. Improve motor skills.

5. Teach functional component skills.

6. Evaluate type of W/C and controls needed (consider consulting OT and research and engineering, if available).

7. Create trunk stability in W/C.

8. Teach W/C skills (consider teaching basic operation of controls in simulator or with W/C motor disengaged).

9. Increase endurance with W/C skills.

10. Determine appropriate W/Cs.

11. Instruct nursing staff, other team members, and significant other in patient's W/C mobility skills.

12. Incorporate skills into daily routine.

13. Evaluate performance in daily routine.

14. Assist patient in problem solving to alleviate difficulties.

Manual Wheelchair Mobility—C5 Quadriplegic

Outcome

1. *Patient demonstrates ability to maneuver independently a manual W/C with oblique projections forward on all smooth level indoor surfaces for approximately 200 to 300 feet before requiring a rest.*

2. Patient demonstrates ability *to assist* and/or direct the maneuvering of manual W/C on all other surfaces.

Components

a. Forward-backward turns

b. Management of all W/C parts (brakes, ramp retarders)

c. Management of doors

d. Indoors:

- all surfaces, tile to carpet
- doorways
- maneuvering in tight places
- elevators
- elevations

e. Outdoors:

- all terrains
- elevations (ramps, curbs, bumps, and cracks in sidewalk)
- crossing streets safely

Considerations

1. Strength, especially:

- shoulder flexors
- elbow flexors
- *shoulder internal rotators*

2. ROM (hips need at least 90 degrees to fit into standard adult W/C)

3. Tone *(increases make trunk stability in W/C difficult and slow speed)*

4. Respiratory status (as it relates to ability to direct care)

5. *Sensory deficits make coordination more difficult*

6. *Obesity*

7. *Age*

8. *Endurance*

9. *Tolerance to vertical*

10. Equipment: What is available to assist?

- type of W/C and accessories
- *back height (increases may increase trunk stability)*
- *recliner W/C (wheel set back 1 inch makes it harder to push)*
- *lighter weight W/C (easier to push)*
- wheels *(pneumatic wheels harder to push if not properly inflated; precision-bearing wheels may be easier to push)*
- *brake extensions*

11. Personality prior to injury:

- How assertive was patient?

12. *Effects of inertia (easier to keep a wheel moving than to start it from a dead stop)*

Process

1. Evaluate motor skills.

2. Evaluate functional component skills:

- head control
- trunk stability in sitting
- balance and equilibrium reactions in sitting
- use of upper extremities in sitting
- *compensatory sensory techniques*
- *skills to compensate for abnormal tone*

3. Improve motor skills.

4. Teach functional component skills.

5. Evaluate type of W/C needed.

6. Create trunk stability in W/C.

7. Consult OT for splinting ideas to aid W/C propulsion.

8. Teach W/C skills.

9. Increase endurance with W/C skills.

10. Determine appropriate W/Cs.

11. Instruct nursing staff, other team members, and significant other in patient's W/C mobility skills.

12. Incorporate skills into daily routine.

13. Evaluate performance in daily routine.

14. Assist patient in problem solving to alleviate difficulties.

Wheelchair Mobility—C6 Quadriplegic

Outcome

1. Patient demonstrates ability to maneuver independently W/C usually *with vertical projections or with plastic-coated handrims and W/C mitts on all smooth level surfaces.*

2. Patient demonstrates ability to assist and/or direct W/C mobility on all other surfaces.

3. *Special consideration may include demonstration of independence with motorized W/C for work and school.*

Components

a. Forward-backward turns

b. Management of all W/C parts (brakes, ramp retarders)

c. Management of doors

d. Indoors:

- all surfaces, tile to carpet
- doorways
- maneuvering in tight places
- elevators
- elevations

e. Outdoors:

- all terrains
- elevations (ramps, curbs, bumps, and cracks in sidewalk)
- crossing streets safely

Considerations

1. Strength, especially:

- shoulder flexors *and extensors*
- elbow flexors
- shoulder internal rotators
- *wrist extensors*

2. ROM:

- *shoulder extension (limitations may decrease speed)*
- hip flexion (90 degrees needed for standard W/C)

3. Tone (increases make trunk stability in W/C difficult and slow speed)

4. Sensory deficits make coordination more difficult

5. Obesity

6. Age

7. Endurance

8. Tolerance to vertical

9. Equipment: What is available to assist?

- back height (increases may increase trunk stability but may also decrease shoulder extension and movement, thus decreasing speed)
- recliner W/C (wheel set back 1 inch makes it harder to push)
- lighter weight W/C (easier to push)
- wheels (pneumatic wheels harder to push if not properly inflated; precision-bearing wheels may be easier to push)
- brake extensions, ramp retarders

10. Personality prior to injury:

- How assertive was patient?

11. Effects of inertia (easier to keep a wheel moving than to start it from a dead stop)

Process

1. Evaluate motor skills.

2. Evaluate functional component skills:

- trunk stability in sitting
- balance and equilibrium reactions in sitting
- use of upper extremities in sitting
- compensatory sensory techniques
- skills to compensate for abnormal tone

3. Improve motor skills.

4. Teach functional component skills.

5. Evaluate type of W/C needed.

6. Create trunk stability in W/C.

7. Teach W/C skills.

8. Increase endurance with W/C skills.

9. Determine appropriate W/Cs.

10. Instruct nursing staff, other team members, and significant other in patient's W/C mobility skills.

11. Incorporate skills into daily routine.

12. Evaluate performance in daily routine.

13. Assist patient in problem solving to alleviate difficulties.

Wheelchair Mobility—C7–8 Quadriplegic

Outcome

1. Patient demonstrates ability to maneuver independently with *or without plastic-coated handrims and W/C mitts on all smooth level surfaces. Maneuvering may be very slow on rough terrain.*

2. Patient demonstrates ability to assist and direct W/C mobility on elevations. (C8 may be independent.)

Components

a. Forward-backward turns

b. *Safe fall out of W/C*

c. Management of all W/C parts (brakes, ramp retarders)

d. Management of doors

e. Indoors:

   - all surfaces, tile to carpet
   - doorways
   - maneuvering in tight places
   - elevators
   - elevations

f. Outdoors:

   - all terrains
   - elevations (ramps, curbs, bumps, and cracks in sidewalk)
   - crossing streets safely

Considerations

1. Strength:

   - *throughout upper extremities*

2. ROM, especially:

   - shoulder extension
   - hip flexion (need WNL for ramps and curbs)

3. Tone (increases make trunk stability in W/C difficult and slow speed)

4. Obesity

5. Age

6. Endurance

7. Equipment: What is available to assist?

   - back height (*may consider decreasing height for increased speed and agility if trunk is stable*)
   - lighter weight W/C (easier to push)
   - wheels (pneumatic wheels harder to push if not properly inflated; precision bearing wheels may be easier to push)
   - ramp retarders

Process

1. Evaluate motor skills.

2. Evaluate functional component skills:

   - trunk stability in sitting
   - balance and equilibrium reactions in sitting
   - use of upper extremities in sitting
   - *wheelies*

3. Improve motor skills.

4. Teach functional component skills.

5. Evaluate type of W/C needed.

6. Teach W/C skills.

7. Increase endurance with W/C skills.

8. Determine appropriate W/Cs.

9. Instruct nursing staff, other team members, and significant other in patient's W/C mobility skills.

10. Incorporate skills into daily routine.

11. Evaluate performance in daily routine.

12. Assist patient in problem solving to alleviate difficulties.

Wheelchair Mobility—T1–L3 Paraplegic

Outcome

1. Patient demonstrates *independent W/C mobility indoors and outdoors in a manual W/C.*

Components

a. Forward-backward turns

b. Safe fall out of W/C

c. Management of all W/C parts (brakes, ramp retarders)

d. Management of doors

e. Indoors:

   - all surfaces, tile to carpet
   - doorways
   - maneuvering in tight places
   - elevators
   - elevations

f. Outdoors:

   - all terrains
   - elevations (ramps, curbs, bumps, and cracks in sidewalk)
   - crossing streets safely

Considerations

1. Strength:

   - throughout upper extremities *and trunk.*

2. ROM, especially:

   - shoulder extension
   - hips (best if within normal limits)

3. Tone

4. Obesity

5. Age

6. Equipment: What is available to assist?

   - *heavy duty durable W/C will be needed (patient usually wears the chair hard)*
   - back height (patient may prefer lower height to increase speed and agility)
   - ramp retarders

Process

1. Evaluate motor skills.

2. Evaluate functional component skills:

   - trunk stability in sitting
   - balance and equilibrium reactions in sitting
   - use of upper extremities in sitting
   - wheelies

3. Improve motor skills.

4. Teach functional component skills.

5. Evaluate type of W/C needed.

6. Teach W/C skills.

7. Increase endurance with W/C skills.

8. Determine appropriate W/Cs.

9. Instruct nursing staff, other team members, and significant other in patient's W/C mobility skills.

10. Incorporate skills into daily routine.

11. Evaluate performance in daily routine.

12. Assist patient in problem solving to alleviate difficulties.

Ambulation

The patient with knee control is often able to use gait patterns similar to those he used before his injury. However, the patterns used will certainly be different for the patient using bilateral KAFOs. Although portions of this chapter will be used to discuss orthotic considerations for a patient with some knee control, most of its focus will be on ambulation considerations for the patient using bilateral KAFOs.

Independent functional ambulation will mean not only that the patient is able to progress forward but also that he is able to climb stairs, curbs, and ramps; don and doff the orthosis; and assume standing.

TO WALK OR NOT TO WALK

Before beginning the subject of gait training, one should perhaps decide whether the therapist and patient should undertake it or not. This is not so much an issue with those patients who obviously will be functional ambulators and not need the use of a W/C, but it becomes much more of an issue with everyone else.

Many therapists will not even begin gait training with a patient unless the patient has, at least, hip flexors. This is because there is a feeling that even if the patients with high-level injuries can walk, they will not be "functional." Walking will take too much energy, and the patient will still use the W/C as the primary means of locomotion. Gait training will not be worth the money and frustration it will cost. Often, even the patient with hip flexors will choose the W/C over walking just because of the time and energy needed to walk. The patient can still go faster and with less energy in a W/C.

This subject of when to gait train or even stand the SCI patient has been debated for years. It is not the intent of this guide to resolve the issue. However, the following paragraphs should give you at least a flavor for some of the historical discussion. (Several representative articles are listed in the bibliography. Refer to these for more detail.)

Some of those in favor of ambulation and standing for the SCI patient present the sort of argument that follows:

1. Most of the body's calcium is found in bone.
2. Any increase in calcium excretion would therefore reflect changes in bone. SCI patients do have an increase in calcium excretion and do have a high incidence of osteoporosis.
3. Increases in calcium excretion have also been postulated as a predisposing factor to *bladder stones* and *ectopic bone*.
4. Pressure can increase bone density and matrix, which encourages more protein to blend with calcium.

5. It is then logical to assume that with ambulation and standing, because of increased pressure on the long bones of the L/E, calcium excretion will be decreased. Therefore, the SCI patient will experience less osteoporosis and ectopic bone formation, fewer bladder stones, and anything else that might occur as a result of calcium imbalances.

There are others, however, who say that ambulation and standing are not enough. A 150-pound man who stands will only produce about 65 pounds of compressive force through the long bones. More pressure is needed to promote bone growth, and this is supplied by muscle contraction. Muscle contraction can provide much more compressive force. In addition it also can provide shearing and torsion forces that may be more significant in increasing bone density than compression is.

There was an interesting study done by Jacqueline Claus-Walker and several physicians at TIRR in the early 1970s. In this study they decided that calcium was more related to duration of paralysis than anything else. Calcium excretion increases during the first ten days post-onset and continues to increase during the next six months. After six months it decreases and levels off to a low normal after about one year.

Furthermore, they felt that increased calcium excretion was not so much related to decreased weight-bearing (and immobilization) as it was to an increase in extracellular fluid volume. They went on to note that the position of the body will influence fluid distribution. Position is ''registered'' by the baroreceptors and transmitted via neural pathways to the central nervous system. In the SCI patient, weight-bearing is often not perceived because the stimulation of the baroreceptors is not able to be transmitted. The neural pathways are not working.

In their study, complete recumbency for three days did *not* increase hypercalciuria in quadriplegics, but calciuria increased 1.5 times in healthy subjects.

So the question still remains: Does one encourage ambulation with one's patients or not? Philosophies will vary on this from one institution to the next. The Rehabilitation Institute of Chicago does not seem to have a fixed and formal policy on the subject. However, the general trend seems to be: *first* provide the patient with the skills needed to be independent from a W/C level and then at least introduce him to ambulation if this is his wish. After all, it is nice to see the world from a standing position once in a while. This does not mean that recommendations for orthotic prescriptions and standing equipment will automatically be made. Temporary equipment is used initially. In the final analysis, whether these recommendations are made to third party payers will be dependent on medical need and functional independence.

However, the feeling at the Rehabilitation Institute of Chicago is that most people psychologically need to prove to themselves that ambulation is not realistic. It's not enough for the medical community to say this. In the past, it was difficult to give patients this opportunity without first purchasing the equipment. However, today there are many commercially available temporary orthotic options. The patient needs to be allowed to use this equipment to discover for himself how much energy and time is needed to get places using both a W/C and orthotics to walk. He can then make his own decision as to which means of locomotion will best suit his needs.

ACHIEVING THE OUTCOME

Energy Expenditure

Normally gait is just a matter of losing and regaining one's balance. For the most part, muscles are used to prevent and control motion rather than to initiate it. Vertical and horizontal oscillations of COG are minimal. All this contributes to decreasing the energy expense during ambulation.

The issue of energy expenditures becomes critical for the SCI patient using bilateral KAFOs. For gait to be effective, energy costs must be minimized.

Some of this cost will be determined by the type of gait pattern the patient is able to use. Depending on the patient and the muscle power present, the four-point or swing-to gait patterns are often the easiest to learn. Skill with these patterns is in addition an asset when it comes to maneuvering in tight and narrow spaces. The swing-through pattern tends to require a little more strength and a greater sense of balance and coordination and may therefore be more difficult to learn. It is, however, generally faster and requires less expenditure of energy if done correctly.

Many of the principles used to conserve energy during normal gait patterns can be applied to the swing-through pattern used by the SCI patient. In this pattern, gait is still a matter of losing and regaining balance. Instructions to patients should incorporate this principle: lean—lift—relax. If instructions start with the word "lift," excessive head movement and trunk flexion are frequently seen. This will create greater vertical oscillations of COG, which increases expenditure of energy. Horizontal oscillations of COG are minimized by maintaining equal stride lengths. This is done by instructing the patient to push with equal strength during the lift and to relax his shoulders simultaneously after the lift. A spreader bar may also be used to facilitate this, particularly if asymmetries in tone and strength are noted.

The push is a critical component of energy expense. If it is too short, the patient will have difficulty with roll-over after heel strike and tend to fall backward. This will obviously cost more energy. If the push is too long, the patient falls forward and is forced to move his crutches quickly forward to catch himself. This robs him of a scheduled time to relax and breaks the rhythm of his pattern. A slow, smooth rhythmic gait pattern will cost less energy.

Some patients prefer longer crutches initially, believing that this will facilitate their lift. When this is done, energy expenditures will be increased because of the increased vertical displacement of the body and the halting gait pattern resulting either from a swing-to gait pattern found when the stride lengths are too short or from a buildup of momentum to the point at which the patient loses control and is forced to stop when the stride lengths are too long.

These are only a few of the many things that should be considered when trying to conserve energy in gait. Close attention to factors that minimize oscillations of COG and the muscle power needed should always be used as a guide to developing a cost-effective gait pattern.

Balance and Forward Progression

Depending on the patient, gait training can take from three to six weeks or longer. It begins in the parallel bars with balancing and weight-shifting activities. If hip extensors are absent, the patient must learn to balance by "hanging" on his Y ligament. Increasing the extension at the hip and low back moves the COG well behind the hip joint, eliminating the need for hip extensors in standing. The upright posture is maintained by the integrity of the Y ligament, which crosses the front of the hip joint and limits further extension at the hip. This makes guarding techniques easy. The therapist stands behind and slightly to the side of the pa-

tient, with one hand at the patient's shoulder and another at his hips. Loss of balance is corrected by pushing the patient's pelvis forward and pulling his shoulders back.

In addition to posture, much of the patient's initial success with balance in standing will depend on how the ankle joints of the orthosis are set. Too much dorsiflexion will cause the patient to fall forward, while too much plantarflexion will push him backward. Increased dorsiflexion on one side will cause him to rotate the pelvis on that side forward and lose his balance to the same side.

The patient should be able to balance in standing without crutches and upper extremity support. If leaning into the crutches is required for balance, the orthosis may not be set correctly. This will force the patient to use more energy just to stand.

Ambulation

After the patient is able to balance in standing, the type of gait pattern the patient will be able to use should be determined. The 4-point gait pattern is perhaps the easiest to learn, especially if the patient has hip flexors, since movement patterns are quite similar to normal walking patterns.

Although the 4-point gait can be useful at times, patients generally do not find it a very useful option. It just takes too much time and energy. Most would prefer either a swing-to or swing-through gait pattern. In the swing-to pattern the patient swings his feet up to but not past the crutches. In the swing-through pattern, the patient swings his feet all the way through and past the crutches. (See previous section for further explanation of this teaching technique.) It is important that the patient learn not to land with the feet in a straight line between his crutches. This destroys the 3-point base of support and makes balancing much more difficult.

Once the patient is comfortable with a progression in the parallel bars, he is ready to move out. How this is accomplished will vary from patient to patient and from therapist to therapist.

Some patients progress immediately from the parallel bars to forearm crutches. Others prefer to take a few extra steps and first practice with one forearm crutch in the parallel bars before they move outside with both. Still others prefer to use a walker next. A walker may give the patient more independence sooner; this may be particularly true with the older patient or the patient with higher level injuries. Once independence is achieved with the walker, he may then progress to fore-arm crutches.

Gait training should include practice on as many different kinds of surfaces as possible (e.g., tile, carpet, sidewalks, gravel), both indoors and outdoors.

Donning and Doffing the Orthosis

Some patients prefer to don and doff the orthosis on a mat or bed in either a long sitting (Figures 10–1a through 10–1c) or sidelying position. Others prefer to remain in a chair (Figures 10–2a through 10–3g). It is usually easier to position the foot in the shoe with knee flexion. Long-handled shoe horns and Velcro closures may also facilitate this procedure.

Stairs

Ascending and descending stairs with bilateral KAFOs (locked in extension) may be accomplished with either a forward or a backward approach. The patient leans and lifts with slight trunk and hip flexion but must quickly return to a position of extension to maintain his balance after landing on the next step. When ascending, the crutches are placed on the step above, but the crutches remain on the same step as the patient when he descends. Strength, timing, and coordination are important to the success of this task. The patient will be most independent if this can be accomplished without the use of railings; however, training usually begins by using one or both railings and then progressing to crutches. Training might also begin by using two- to three-inch steps and then progress to a higher step. Stair "lips" may make this activity more difficult. The patient tends to catch the toes of his shoes on these and trip. It may be best to approach these stairs backward.

With increased knee control, climbing stairs requires less energy and other approaches may be available. The training process, however, is similar. The patient usually starts with a two- to three-inch step, using one or both railings, and progresses to the higher step using only his assistive devices (e.g., crutches, canes).

Some patients find walking up and down stairs too difficult and energy consuming and would rather sit down and scoot up or down on their buttocks. This is certainly a reasonable option, although it can be a little rough on the skin. Skin should be watched more closely for signs of pressure sore development.

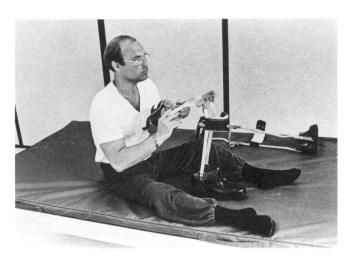

Figure 10–1a Patient dons KAFO from long sitting position. Good long sitting balance is required.

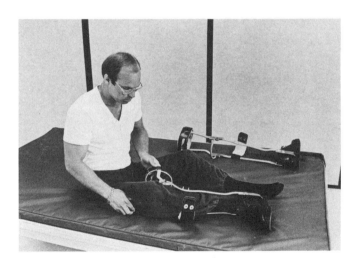

Figure 10–1b

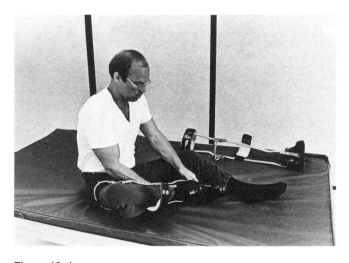

Figure 10–1c

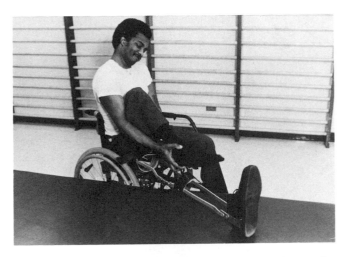

Figure 10–2a Patient dons KAFOs from a W/C using the mat for additional support.

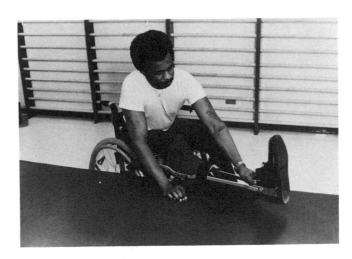

Figure 10–2b

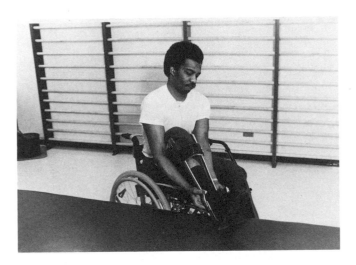

Figure 10–2c

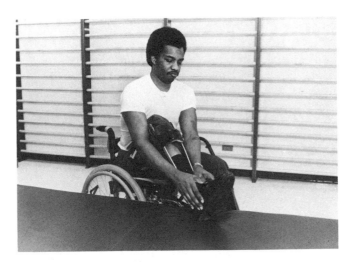

Figure 10–2d

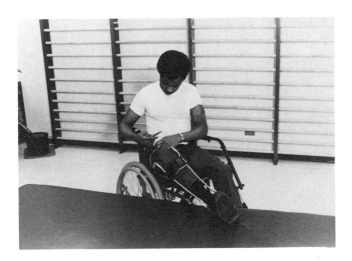

Figure 10–2e

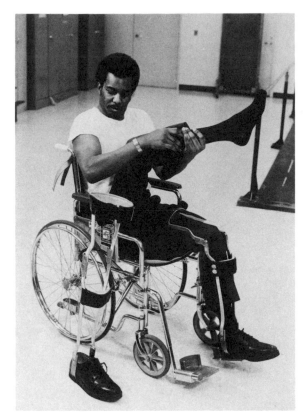

Figure 10–3a Patient dons KAFOs from W/C. Note flexibility.

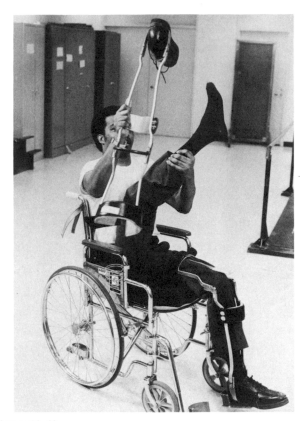

Figure 10–3b

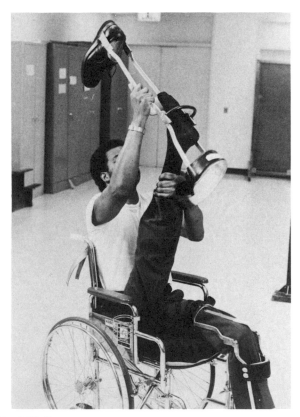

Figure 10–3c

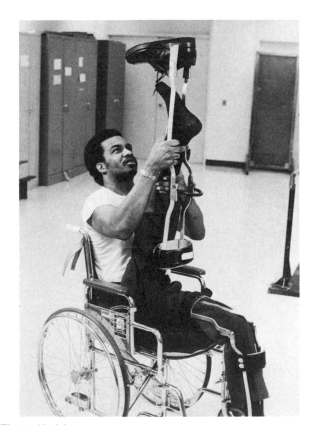

Figure 10–3d

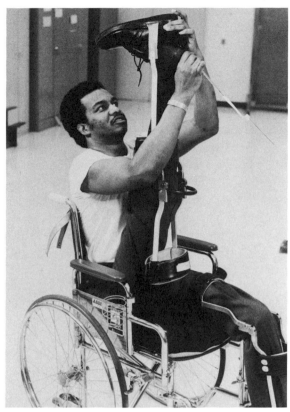

Figure 10–3e

Curbs

After a patient is comfortable climbing and descending stairs, he should then be introduced to curbs. The techniques used are similar to those used on the stairs. One should start with a one-inch or two-inch curb and progress to six-inch curbs. With smaller curbs, the patient may be able to ascend, keeping both crutches on the lower level; with higher curbs, the crutches will need to be on the higher level.

Ramps

The patient should be taught how to approach a variety of ramps. The methods used will vary, depending on the degree of incline, the surface of the incline, and the patient. On slight inclines, the patient using bilateral KAFOs will still be able to use a swing-through pattern; however, the activity is easier if he uses a shorter stride length ascending the incline and a longer stride length on the descent. Steeper inclines may require a swing-to pattern. All possible angles of approach should be considered: forward, backward, sideways, and diagonally. As with anything else, ramps require

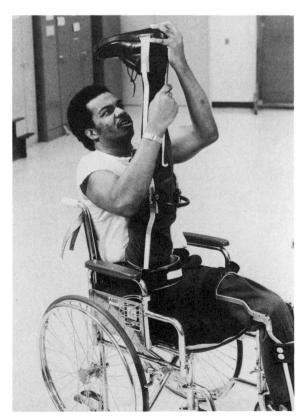

Figure 10–3f

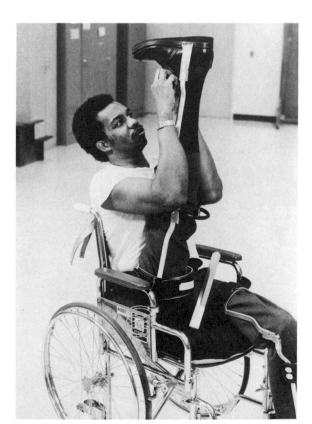

Figure 10–3g

experimentation on the part of the therapist and patient to determine the best approach.

Assumption of Standing from a Chair

Two methods are available (Figures 10–4a through 10–5d):

1. Crutches are placed on either side of the W/C and knees are locked. The patient scoots to the edge of the chair and crosses one leg over the other. If bail locks are used, he may need to balance the heel of one foot on the toe of the other to prevent knee unlocking. He then pivots around and pushes to standing, facing the chair. Putting the desk armrests of the W/C on backward or raising the height of the adjustable armrests can make this activity easier. After his feet are flat and he is well balanced, he reaches for one crutch and then the other. Because stepping backward is usually not easily done, moving away from the W/C once standing may be the most difficult aspect of this approach. However, if moving backward is not an option, most are able to side-step or circle around away from the chair.

2. To assume standing coming out of the chair forward, the patient again scoots to the edge of the chair and locks his knees. The crutches are placed perpendicular to the floor just behind the casters. The patient tucks his head and does a quick forceful push down, lifting himself to a vertical position. He must land with his feet flat and immediately extend at the head, trunk, and hip. This method is usually more difficult and generally requires more balance and coordination. It is, however, faster.

The reverse of these techniques is used to return to sitting. Unless bail locks are used, it is difficult to use a straight back approach to return to sitting. In those instances, it may be easier to use the first option, facing the W/C initially and twisting back down to sitting.

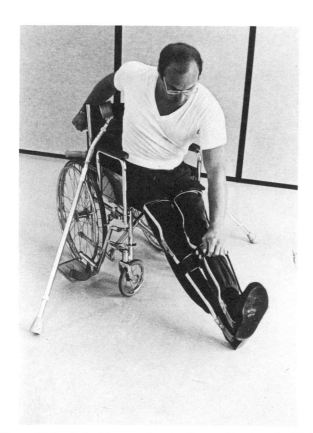

Figure 10–4a Patient is assuming standing position from the W/C.

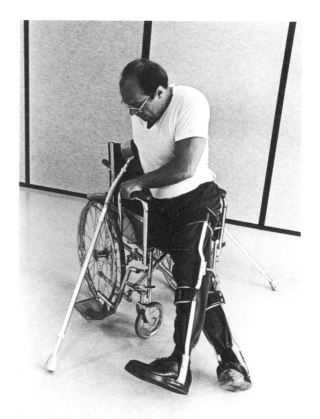

Figure 10–4b

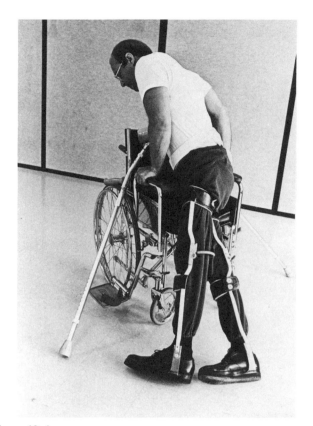

Figure 10–4c

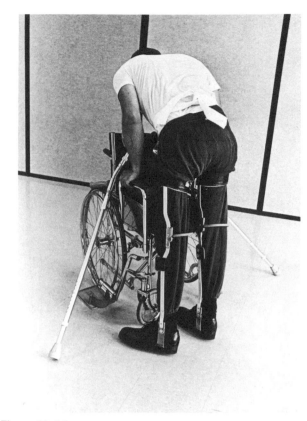

Figure 10–4d

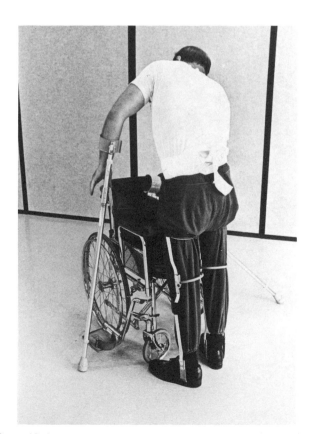

Figure 10–4e

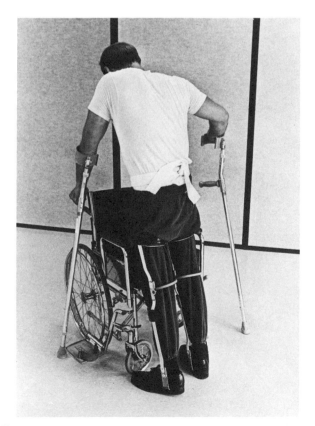

Figure 10–4f

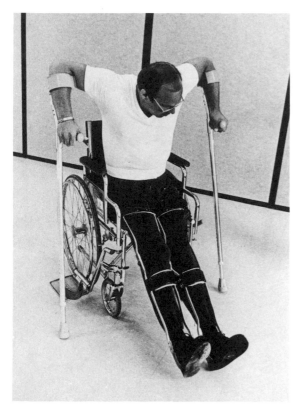

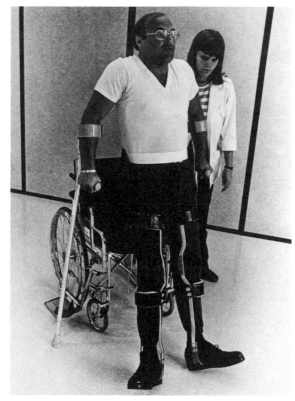

Figure 10–5a Patient is assuming standing position from W/C. Note the head and upper trunk flexion. This will place the latissimus dorsi and triceps on stretch, facilitating a stronger lift.

Figure 10–5b

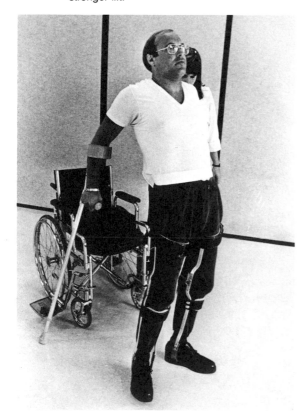

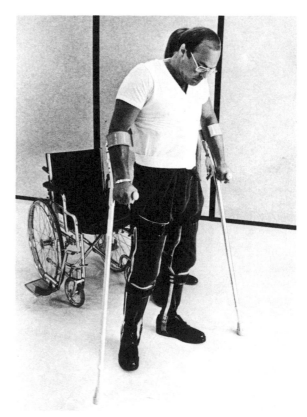

Figure 10–5c

Figure 10–5d

Falling

Unfortunately, one must assume that a patient will fall regardless of how independent he may be. The patient with hip and knee control still has many equilibrium reactions available to him, but without this control he has many less balance options and is frequently unable to regain his balance once he starts to fall.

For this reason, the person using bilateral KAFOs independently should be taught to fall forward safely (Figure 10–6). This can be frightening. Much support and guidance need to be given initially. The patient simply releases his crutches, throws them clear of his body, and reaches for the ground. He should land with flexed elbows and slowly lower himself down.

Assumption of Standing from the Floor

If a patient must learn how to fall to the ground, it follows that he must also learn how to assume standing from the ground. This is perhaps the most difficult to learn for the patient using bilateral KAFO. Again, he has two options:

1. Lying on his stomach, the patient places his crutches so that the cuffs are about knee level. Placement will vary a little, depending on the patient.

He then pushes up to the plantegrade position and either pulls his feet up to his hands or walks back on his hands until his feet are flat. With a good head tuck, pulling the legs up to the feet can sometimes be easier and quicker. Walking the hands back is a slower process and may require more strength and endurance. If the patient chooses to walk his hands back, he may find it easier to do if his feet are initially placed near a wall so they do not slide. If hamstrings are tight, starting with the legs spread farther apart into abduction may be easier.

Once in the plantegrade position, the patient reaches for one crutch, gets his balance with this either by resting the grip on his shoulder or by holding onto the grip, and reaches for the other crutch, pushing the rest of the way to standing (Figures 10–7a through 10–8d). Initially, the therapist may need to provide moderate to maximum support at the hips while the patient attempts to pick up the crutches and position them. This method requires adequate ROM, much strength and endurance, and good coordination and balance.

2. The patient first transfers into a chair and then assumes standing. (See section on floor to W/C transfers in Chapter 8.)

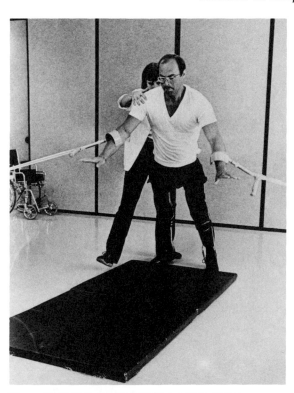

Figure 10–6 Patient with KAFOs practices falling.

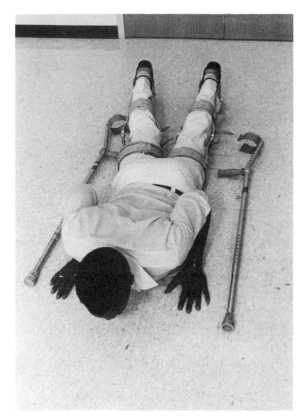

Figure 10–7a Patient is assuming standing from the floor. Note position of crutches.

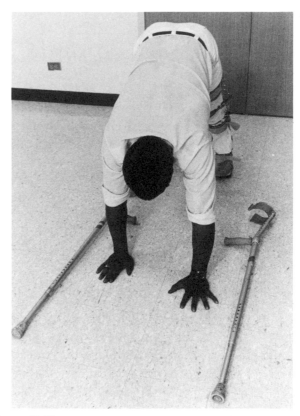

Figure 10–7b

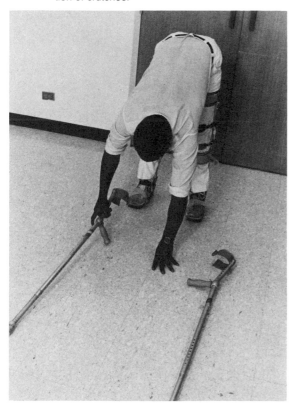

Figure 10–7c

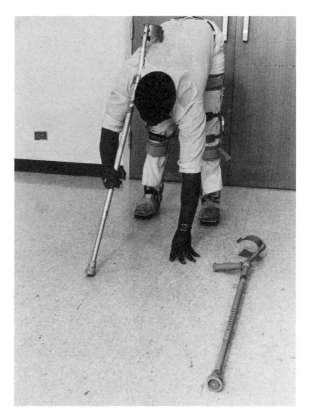

Figure 10–7d Note position of crutch. This can provide a stable position, but to maintain it for a long period of time could cause a brachial plexus injury.

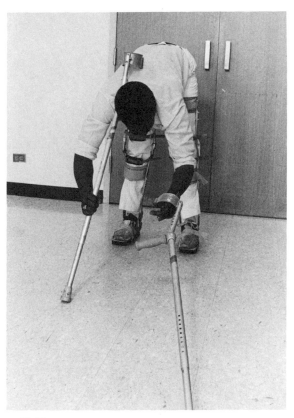

Figure 10–7e

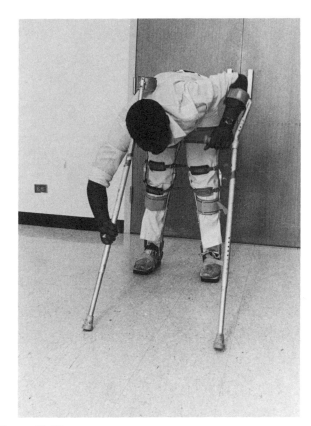

Figure 10–7f

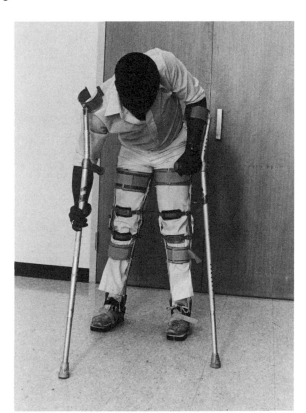

Figure 10–7g

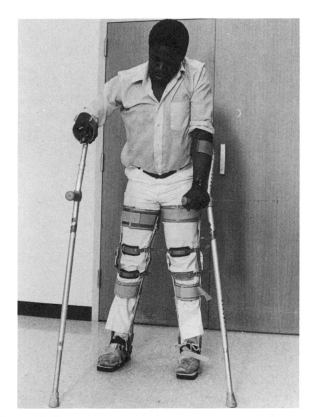

Figure 10–7h

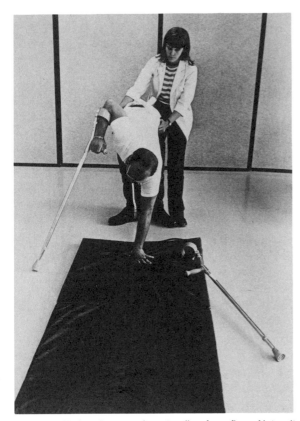

Figure 10–8a Patient is assuming standing from floor. Note alternative use of first crutch.

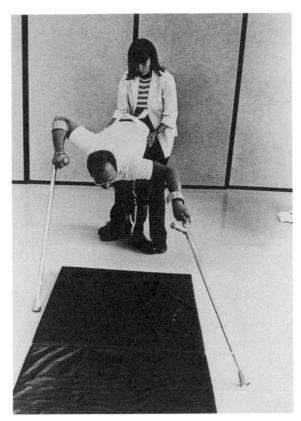

Figure 10–8b

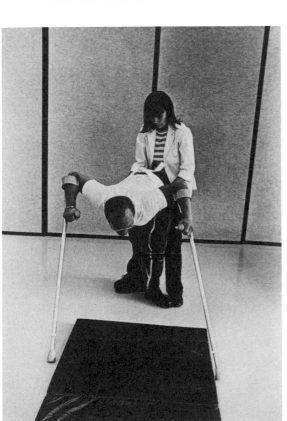

Figure 10–8c

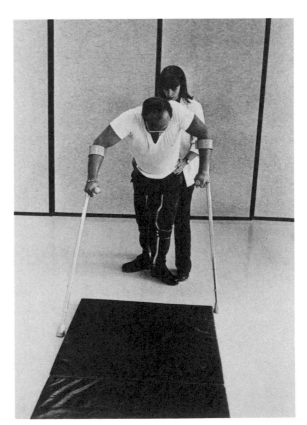

Figure 10–8d

EQUIPMENT OPTIONS

Depending on the level of injury, lower extremity orthoses can offer many options for the SCI patient. A few of the advantages and disadvantages of some of these orthoses are listed in Tables 10–1 and 10–2. Neither the list of devices nor the listed considerations of these devices is meant to be inclusive.

TABLE 10–1   Knee-Ankle-Foot Orthosis (KAFO)

Craig-Scott KAFO	Conventional KAFO
This orthosis was designed in 1960 for the patient using a swing-to gait pattern. It is not so much the components used but the combination of these parts that distinguishes it from the conventional KAFO. Some components that help define this orthosis are: a transverse sole plate and extended longitudinal plate, a double stirrup with a strut, a special shoe wedge that extends almost the entire length of the shoe, a cushioned heel, ankle joints fixed in 10° of dorsiflexion, knee joints offset ½ inch posterior to the anatomical knee joint, a bail locking system, and a solid pretibial band.	This orthosis is usually made with double-action ankle joints and an extended steel shank. Knee joints are normally not offset posteriorly, and a variety of different locking systems is available for this joint. The tibial band encloses the calf, and the posterior thigh band is traditionally higher than that used in the Craig-Scott.
May provide more stability.	May provide more mobility.
Fixed ankle joints may improve balance.	It is lighter (by approximately 2 lbs.).
Cushioned heel may provide a softer landing and improved roll-over.	More alternative component parts are available.
It is easier to don and doff.	4-point gait may be easier, depending on the ankle adjustment (more difficult with the Craig-Scott because of the fixed ankle and inflexible shoe).
Offset knee easier to unlock.	Assumption of standing from floor may be easier (fixed ankle joint and inflexible shoe of Craig-Scott makes this difficult).
Decreased height of posterior calf band may allow increased hyperextension at hip.	There is less tibial pressure (Craig-Scott has no posterior closure below the knee, so it can slide forward on the leg in transfers and can create more rubbing on the tibia).
Decreased height of medial upright may decrease adductor stimulation.	It provides more stability around the knee joint (with lax ligaments, the patient may develop more instability with the Craig-Scott).
Training time may be decreased through added stability and balance.	It is less expensive.
Has a decreased hardware effect.	Progression from KAFO to AFO is easier in that the patient can train with the knees unlocked using ball-bearing retainers.

Polypropylene KAFOs have been used occasionally. They seem to be most appropriate when the patient has minimal increases in tone and minimal sensation losses. The orthosis can be lighter than the conventional or the Craig-Scott KAFO, but this will depend on how much metal needs to be used for the joints. If both knee and ankle joints are required, the weight of the orthosis is approximately the same as the others. Because of the precise fit, patients often complain that it is hot and uncomfortable in sitting. Edema is harder to accommodate, and there may be increased potential for pressure areas.

TABLE 10–2   Ankle-Foot Orthosis (AFO)

Double-Action AFO with Extended Steel Shank	Polypropylene AFO
Ankle joint can accommodate many changes in position.	It is lighter.
Proprioceptive feedback may be increased due to increased weight.	It tends to be more definitive because adjustments available at the ankle joint are minimal. However, some function changes can be made by adjusting the shoe heel height.
Fluctuating edema is more easily accommodated.	
Shoes cannot be changed unless UCB/NYU shoe insert is used.	Flexibility of the orthosis can be increased by cutting back the trim lines around the ankle.
	It can be more cosmetic because it can be worn in many different shoes. (Shoes should be about one-half size larger than what one would ordinarily wear and should have similar heel heights.)
	Plastic does not absorb perspiration, and this can make wearing the shoes uncomfortable.
	Abrupt temperature changes may cause cracking.
	Fluctuating edema is difficult to accommodate.

The single-action AFO has some limited value. It can act as a dorsiflexion aid and is able to limit the amount of plantarflexion. However, knee control with this orthosis is difficult because of its inability to limit the dorsiflexion motion at the ankle. If the patient's neurological picture has stabilized and ankle control is all that is needed, the single-action AFO may be a good choice.

FINAL COMMENT

In addition to the above-noted considerations, all orthotic decisions should take into account the orthotist and his expertise. Some orthotists, for instance, are just not as experienced working with polypropylene as are others. If no other orthotist is available, it might be beneficial to use the more conventional orthosis.

Ambulation—T6–8 Paraplegic

Outcome

1. Patient demonstrates ability to ambulate independently in parallel bars with bilateral KAFOs using swing-to gait pattern.

2. Patient demonstrates ability to ambulate usually with supervision using bilateral KAFOs and a walker for short distances. (Patient may require assistance to assume standing outside the bars.)

Components

a. Donning and doffing orthosis

b. Moving forward, backward, sideways, and turning to both right and left

c. Maneuvering in narrow spaces

d. Assumption of standing and return to sitting

e. Ability to fall safely.

Considerations

1. Strength, especially:
   - upper extremities
   - trunk

2. ROM, especially:
   - hip extension
   - knee extension
   - ankle dorsiflexion

3. Tone

4. Coordination

5. Endurance (skill requires high endurance levels)

6. Body build, weight, proportions

7. Age

8. Fear of falling

9. Equipment: What is available to assist?
   - orthosis (provides varying degrees of stability and mobility)
   - spreader bar (may assist with foot placement, especially in instances where asymmetries in tone are noted)

Process

1. Evaluate motor skills.

2. Evaluate functional component skills:
   - ability to lean into Y ligament at hip and maintain balance both with and without upper extremity support
   - weight shift in standing
   - ability to stabilize trunk in standing and move upper extremities
   - ability to stabilize trunk in standing, lift, and move lower extremities
   - foot placement

3. Improve motor skills.

4. Evaluate and determine appropriate orthosis and assistive devices.

5. Teach functional component skills.

6. Teach ambulation skills.

7. Increase endurance.

8. Instruct nursing staff, other team members, and significant others in ambulation skills.

9. Incorporate skills into daily routine.

10. Evaluate performance in daily routine.

11. Assist patient in problem solving to alleviate difficulties.

Ambulation—T9–12 Paraplegic

Outcome

1. Patient demonstrates ability to ambulate independently with bilateral KAFOs, *using either a walker or forearm crutches with a swing-to or swing-through gait pattern on level surfaces.*

2. *Patient demonstrates ability to ambulate with supervision on elevations and rough terrain.*

Components

a. Donning and doffing orthosis

b. Moving forward, backward, sideways, and turning to both right and left

c. All surfaces—smooth to rough and uneven (sand, grass, carpets, tile)

d. Maneuvering in narrow spaces

e. *Elevations:*
   - *stairs*
   - *ramps*
   - *curbs: 2–inch, 4–inch, and 6–inch*

f. *Elevators*

g. *Escalators*

h. Standing to sitting to standing from all chairs

i. *Ability to fall safely*

j. *Ability to assume standing from floor*

Considerations

1. Strength, especially:
   - upper extremities
   - trunk
   - *quadratus lumborum*

2. ROM, especially:
   - hip extension
   - knee extension
   - ankle dorsiflexion

3. Tone

4. Coordination

5. Endurance (skill requires high endurance levels)

6. Body build, weight, proportions

7. Age

8. Fear of falling

9. Equipment: What is available to assist?
   - orthosis (provides varying degrees of stability and mobility)
   - spreader bar (may assist with foot placement, especially in instances where asymmetries in tone are noted)

Process

1. Evaluate motor skills.

2. Evaluate functional component skills:
   - ability to lean into Y ligament at hip and maintain balance both with and without upper extremity support
   - weight shift in standing
   - ability to stabilize trunk in standing and move upper extremities
   - ability to stabilize trunk in standing, lift, and move lower extremities
   - foot placement

3. Improve motor skills.

4. Evaluate and determine appropriate orthosis and assistive devices.

5. Teach functional component skills.

6. Teach ambulation skills.

7. Increase endurance.

8. Instruct nursing staff, other team members, and significant others in ambulation skills.

9. Incorporate skills into daily routine.

10. Evaluate performance in daily routine.

11. Assist patient in problem solving to alleviate difficulties.

Ambulation—T12–L3 Paraplegic

Outcome

1. Patient demonstrates ability to ambulate independently with bilateral KAFOs, using forearm crutches with a swing-to, swing-through, or *four-point gait pattern on level surfaces and elevations.*

Components

a. Donning and doffing orthosis

b. Moving forward, backward, sideways, and turning to both right and left

c. All surfaces—smooth to rough and uneven (sand, grass, carpets, tile)

d. Maneuvering in narrow spaces

e. Elevations:
   - stairs
   - ramps
   - curbs: 2–inch, 4–inch, and 6–inch

f. Elevators

g. Escalators

h. Standing to sitting to standing from all chairs

i. Ability to fall safely

j. Ability to assume standing from floor

Considerations

1. Strength, especially:
   - upper extremities
   - trunk
   - *hip flexors*

2. ROM, especially:
   - hip extension
   - knee extension
   - ankle dorsiflexion

3. Tone

4. Coordination

5. Endurance (skill requires high endurance levels)

6. Body build, weight, proportions

7. Age

8. Fear of falling

9. Equipment: What is available to assist?
   - orthosis (provides varying degrees of stability and mobility)
   - spreader bar (may assist with foot placement, especially in instances where asymmetries in tone are noted)

Process

1. Evaluate motor skills.

2. Evaluate functional component skills:
   - standing balance both with and without upper extremity support
   - weight shift in standing
   - ability to stabilize trunk in standing and move upper extremities
   - ability to stabilize trunk in standing and move lower extremities
   - foot placement

3. Improve motor skills.

4. Evaluate and determine appropriate orthosis and assistive devices.

5. Teach functional component skills.

6. Teach ambulation skills.

7. Increase endurance.

8. Instruct nursing staff, other team members, and significant others in ambulation skills.

9. Incorporate skills into daily routine.

10. Evaluate performance in daily routine.

11. Assist patient in problem solving to alleviate difficulties.

Ambulation—L4–5 Paraplegic

Outcome

1. Patient demonstrates *ability to ambulate independently with bilateral AFOs and forearm crutches or canes, using a four-point or two-point gait pattern on level surfaces and elevations.*

Components

a. Donning and doffing orthosis

b. Moving forward, backward, sideways, and turning to both right and left

c. All surfaces—smooth to rough and uneven (sand, grass, carpets, tile)

d. Maneuvering in narrow spaces

e. Elevations:

- stairs
- ramps
- curbs: 2–inch, 4–inch, and 6–inch

f. Elevators

g. Escalators

h. Standing to sitting to standing from all chairs

i. Ability to assume standing from floor

Considerations

1. Strength, especially:

- *knee flexors*
- *knee extensors*
- *hip musculature*

2. ROM, especially:

- knee extension
- ankle dorsiflexion

3. Tone

4. Obesity

5. Age

6. Equipment: What is available to assist?

- orthosis (provide varying degrees of stability and mobility)

Process

1. Evaluate motor skills.

2. Evaluate functional component skills:

- standing balance both with and without upper extremity support
- weight shift in standing both side to side and forward and back
- *knee control*
- foot placement

3. Improve motor skills.

4. Evaluate and determine appropriate orthosis and assistive devices.

5. Teach functional component skills.

6. Teach ambulation skills.

7. Increase endurance.

8. Instruct nursing staff, other team members, and significant others in ambulation skills.

9. Incorporate skills into daily routine.

10. Evaluate performance in daily routine.

11. Assist patient in problem solving to alleviate difficulties.

Self-ROM

Able-bodied persons usually move their joints through their available ranges many times during the course of a day. The SCI patient, however, is moving less. Daily activities may not require full ROM at all the joints, leaving room for tightness and contractures to develop. Increases in tone can further complicate the picture. If tightness is allowed to develop, ADL can become more limited than it might already be. Many patients need to have assistance to do their ROM. However, there are also many who are able to do this on their own.

ACHIEVING THE OUTCOME

Teaching self-ROM is fairly straightforward. Since, for the most part, good upper extremity strength is required to accomplish this skill, the primary concern is ROM of the lower extremities and trunk. The patient should be taught how to stretch into all available motions in the lower extremities. Activities to maintain trunk flexibility should also be included.

Even though normal strength is present, occasional tightness or a tendency toward tightness is often noted in some upper extremity motions, particularly horizontal abduction and shoulder flexion. Any self-ROM techniques should include activities to compensate for this.

Careful attention to good posture and normal alignment of body parts will ensure that the appropriate muscles are being stretched. Remember to teach the patients the concepts. Do not just give them a cookbook of activities to do. Patients need to learn to generalize from one situation to the next. Therapists should help patients incorporate as many of their ROM needs as possible into functional activities. In this way, patients will be able to avoid things like inadvertently over-stretching their low back in an attempt to put on shoes and pants. Picture handouts are always helpful. Some examples follow.

Hip external rotation and abduction can be stretched in a long-sitting position by bending the knee and rocking it out to the side (Figures 11–1 and 11–2). Hip internal rotation and adduction can be stretched in this same position if the knee is then rocked in, past the midline (Figure 11–3).

If the patient presents with lumbar flexion and a posteriorly rotated pelvis, ROM should be done with the back well supported maintaining a neutral vertebral column and pelvis. This approach can also be used with the patient who has poor sitting balance (Figures 11–4 and 11–5).

An alternate way of stretching hip abduction and adduction is illustrated in Figures 11–6a through 11–7b.

Hip and Knee Flexion with Abduction/External Rotation and Adduction/Internal Rotation

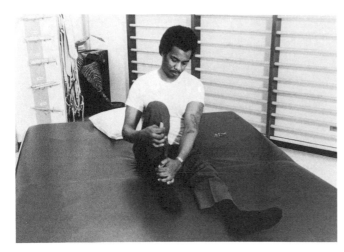

Figure 11–1 Patient is using long sitting position to provide hip ROM. (Also shown in Figures 11–2 and 11–3.)

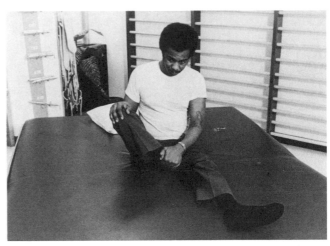

Figure 11–2 Hip and knee flexion with abduction and external rotation.

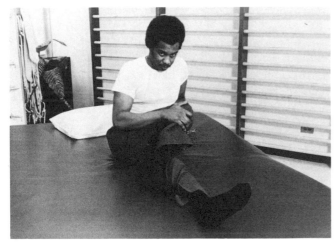

Figure 11–3 Hip and knee flexion with adduction and internal rotation.

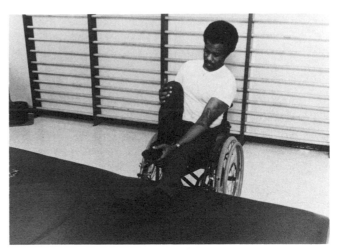

Figure 11–4 Patient is using the W/C to support his back while giving ROM to his hips. (Also shown in Figure 11–5.)

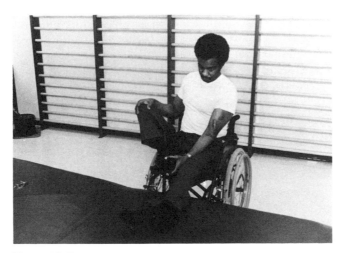

Figure 11–5

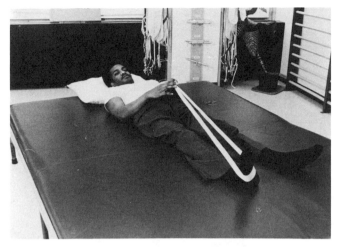

Figure 11–6a Patient, in supine position, uses loop to stretch into hip abduction. (Also shown in Figure 11–6b.)

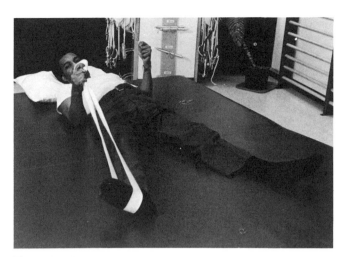

Figure 11–6b

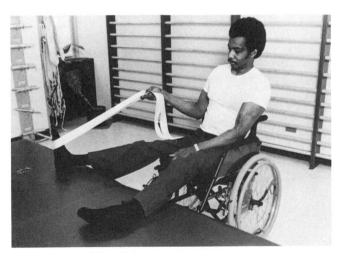

Figure 11–7a Patient uses W/C to support his back while he stretches into hip abduction using a loop. (Also shown in Figure 11–7b.)

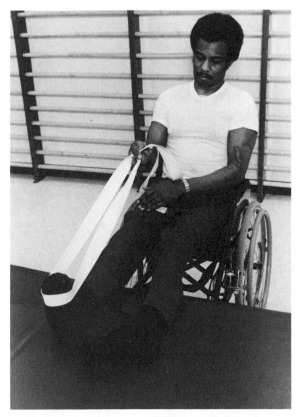

Figure 11–7b Patient brings leg back into midline.

Hip flexion combined with knee extension can be stretched in a supine position with or without using a loop (Figures 11–8a through 11–9c).

Note: if a patient has a flexible back, a towel roll might be placed in the low back. This will block the pelvis from rotating posteriorly and encourage stretching of the hamstrings rather than the low back.

Hip Flexion with Knee Extension

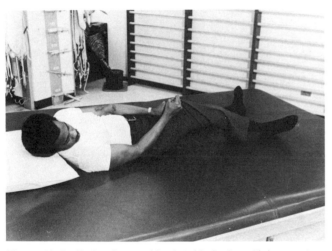

Figure 11–8a Patient is stretching into hip flexion with knee extension.

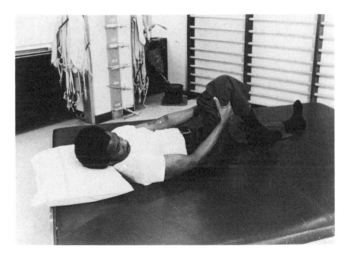

Figure 11–8b

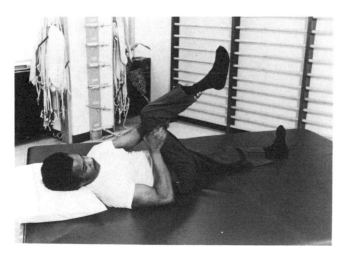

Figure 11–8c

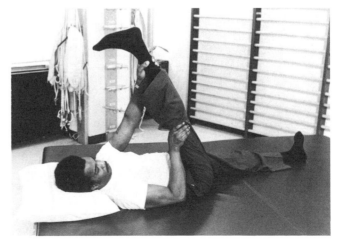

Figure 11–8d

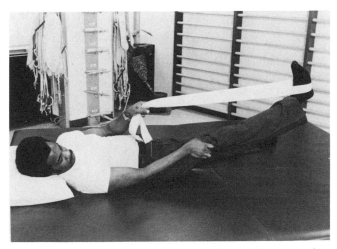

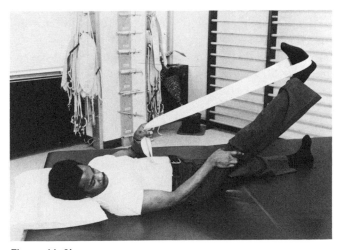

Figure 11–9a Patient is stretching into hip flexion with knee extension using a loop. (Also shown in Figures 11–9b and 11–9c.)

Figure 11–9b

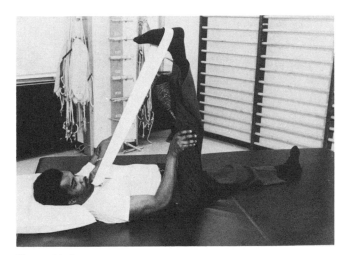

Figure 11–9c

There are many ways to stretch into ankle dorsiflexion. The primary concern is to localize the stretch. The patient in Figure 11–10 is attempting to prevent overstretching of the forefoot by placing more emphasis on the push of the bottom hand on the heel. The pull with the top hand at the toes is minimal. The patient in Figure 11–11 has placed a towel roll under the knee to prevent overstretching of the knee joint and capsule, but his use of a loop may overstretch the forefoot. The patient in Figure 11–12 uses his shoe to provide a better heel grip reducing the tendency to overstretch the forefoot with the loop.

Ankle Dorsiflexion

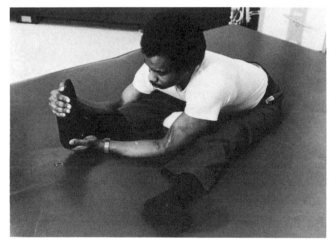

Figure 11–10 Patient is stretching into dorsiflexion in a long sitting position.

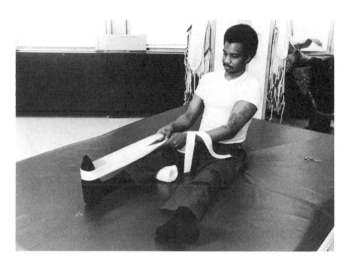

Figure 11–11 Patient is using a loop to stretch into dorsiflexion.

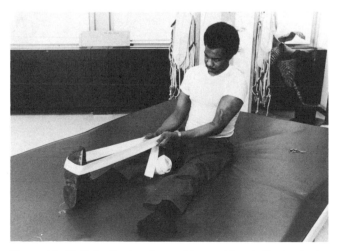

Figure 11–12 Patient's shoe is used to provide a better heel grip, giving a better stretch to the plantarflexor muscles.

The stretching can be done either on a mat or bed or in the W/C as is seen in Figures 11–13 and 11–14.

If tight hamstrings are present, stretching into dorsiflexion with hip and knee flexion will prevent overstretching of the back (Figure 11–15). The quadriplegic patient may also use this position to stretch into dorsiflexion with his forearm (Figure 11–16).

Note: Since the gastrocnemius muscle is a two-joint muscle, this position will not provide as much stretch as a position with the knee extended.

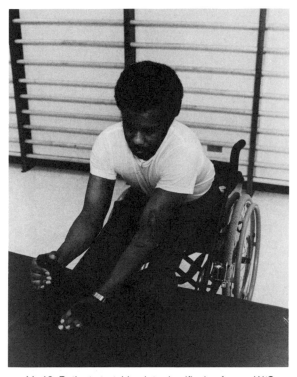

Figure 11–13 Patient stretching into dorsiflexion from a W/C.

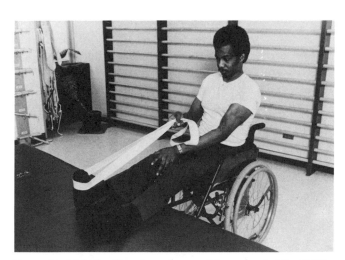

Figure 11–14 Patient is using a loop and the support of the W/C to stretch into dorsiflexion.

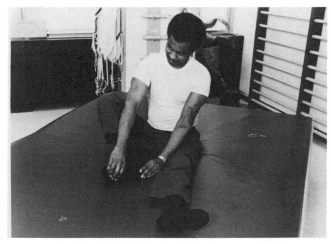

Figure 11–15 Patient is using hip and knee flexion to stretch into dorsiflexion.

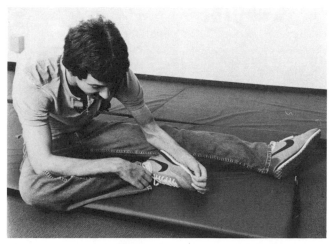

Figure 11–16 A quadriplegic patient can stretch ankle plantarflexors with his forearm.

Hip Extension

The methods shown in Figures 11–17 and 11–18 can be used to stretch into hip extension. If lordosis is present, pillows should be used under the hips to place the pelvis in neutral rotation (Figure 11–17). If the patient presents with a kyphosis and lumbar flexion, no pillows should be used under the hips (Figure 11–18).

While these methods can maintain hip extension and perhaps stretch some mild contractures, the Thomas position is probably a better position in which to stretch the hip flexors. In this position gravity can be used to assist the stretch.

The patient should lie supine with one leg hanging off the front of the table, which should hit the leg at the mid thigh. The opposite leg is pulled up into full hip and knee flexion. This will lock the pelvis and ensure that stretch takes place across the hip joint and prevent the low back from arching.

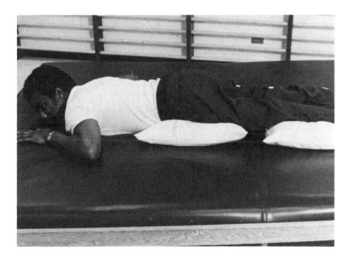

Figure 11–17 Patient with lordosis stretching into hip extension using pillows.

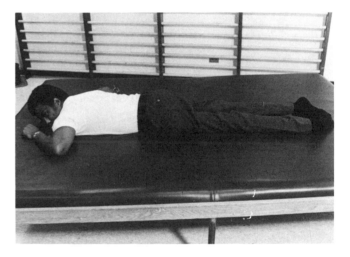

Figure 11–18 Patient with a kyphosis should use this position to stretch into hip extension. No pillow should be used.

Self-ROM—C6 Quadriplegic

Outcome

1. Patient demonstrates ability to assist or perform parts of his ROM.

Components

a. All available motions at each individual joint

Considerations

1. Medical complications

   - Ectopic bone formation may significantly decrease ROM in some joints, preventing patient from assuming postures that would allow him to range other joints independently.

2. Tone

3. Age

4. Obesity

5. ADL independence may determine techniques used.

Process

1. Evaluate motor skills.

2. Evaluate functional component skills:

   - rolling
   - balance and equilibrium reactions on elbows
   - balance and equilibrium reactions in sitting, both with and without upper extremity support

3. Improve motor skills.

4. Teach functional component skills.

5. Teach self-ROM techniques (coordinate with OT and nursing).

6. Observe and evaluate patient's return demonstration.

7. Incorporate skills into daily routine.

8. As patient becomes more independent with other ADL skills, reevaluate the need for formal ROM to each individual joint. For instance, patient may be receiving adequate ROM to shoulders during dressing, good hip flexion during transfers, and good hip extension with prone activities.

9. Discontinue formal ROM to individual joints as appropriate and incorporate ranging into functional daily activities.

10. Evaluate performance in daily routine.

11. If formal ROM to individual joints has been discontinued, reevaluate ROM at all joints to ensure that no motions are being lost.

Self-ROM—C7–8 Quadriplegic

Outcome

1. Patient demonstrates ability to perform self-ROM independently.

Components

a. All available motions at each individual joint

Considerations

1. Medical complications:

   - Ectopic bone formation may significantly decrease ROM in some joints, preventing patient from assuming postures that would allow him to independently range other joints.

2. Tone

3. Age

4. Obesity

5. ADL independence may determine techniques used.

Process

1. Evaluate motor skills.

2. Evaluate functional component skills:

   - rolling
   - balance and equilibrium reactions on elbows
   - balance and equilibrium reactions in sitting, both with and without upper extremity support

3. Improve motor skills.

4. Teach functional component skills.

5. Teach self-ROM techniques (coordinate with OT and nursing).

6. Observe and evaluate patient's return demonstration.

7. Incorporate skills into daily routine.

8. As patient becomes more independent with other ADL skills, reevaluate the need for formal ROM to each individual joint. For instance, patient may be receiving adequate ROM to shoulders during dressing, good hip flexion during transfers, and good hip extension with prone activities.

9. Discontinue formal ROM to individual joints as appropriate and incorporate ranging into functional daily activities.

10. Evaluate performance in daily routine.

11. If formal ROM to individual joints has been discontinued, reevaluate ROM at all joints to ensure that no motions are being lost.

Self-ROM—Paraplegic

Outcome

1. Patient demonstrates ability to perform self-ROM independently.

Components

a. All available motions at each individual joint

Considerations

1. Medical complications:
   - Ectopic bone formation may significantly decrease ROM in some joints, preventing patient from assuming postures that would allow him to independently range other joints.

2. Tone

3. Age

4. Obesity

5. ADL independence may determine techniques used.

Process

1. Evaluate motor skills.

2. Evaluate functional component skills:
   - rolling
   - balance and equilibrium reactions on elbows
   - balance and equilibrium reactions in sitting, both with and without upper extremity support

3. Improve motor skills.

4. Teach functional component skills.

5. Teach self-ROM techniques (coordinate with OT and nursing).

6. Observe and evaluate patient's return demonstration.

7. Incorporate skills into daily routine.

8. As patient becomes more independent with other ADL skills, reevaluate the need for formal ROM to each individual joint. For instance, patient may be receiving adequate ROM to shoulders during dressing, good hip flexion during transfers, and good hip extension with prone activities.

9. Discontinue formal ROM to individual joints as appropriate and incorporate ranging into functional daily activities.

10. Evaluate performance in daily routine.

11. If formal ROM to individual joints has been discontinued, reevaluate ROM at all joints to ensure that no motions are being lost.

Discharge Planning

Mat programs and ADL training teach a person how to move in bed, transfer, and ambulate; but this is only *part* of what is necessary to reenter life's mainstream. What accessibility problems will exist with use of prescribed equipment? How will mobility skills be maintained and/or upgraded? Are home programs necessary? What should be included in these programs? What should be included in family teaching?

HOME PROGRAMS

Home programs do have a place in discharge planning. However, in order to be effective, some practical and realistic planning has to occur. After all, how many people actually include an hour of exercise into their daily schedules? The disabled individual already has to spend more time with his daily care needs than the able-bodied population. Why burden him with another hour of exercise or the stress of finding someone to assist him with exercising when the exercises may not be needed or when the assistant may be impossible to find? Therefore, before any programs can be developed, several basic questions need to be considered:

- *What will the patient be able to do when discharged?* Will he be doing transfers independently? How will he do them? Will he be ambulatory? Will he reach his optimum levels of independence before discharge, or will he need to continue upgrading on his own at home?

- *What will the patient need to maintain his ADL skills?* At this point, we are considering motor skills: ROM, strength, balance, respiratory skills, and so on. What are the ROM and strength requirements for the patient to perform independent transfers? Even if the patient will be basically ADL dependent, these areas still require consideration. Someone will still need to move him, transfer him, and dress him. A certain amount of range and flexibility is still required. The easier a person is to move, the more likely it is that he will be moved.

- *What will the patient need to maintain his health?* The primary issues here are skin integrity and respiratory status. In both of these areas, positional changes are important. Without these positional changes, the likelihood of pressure sores and pneumonia increases. Will the patient's daily routine on discharge include positional changes?

- *What skills will the patient be able to maintain just by completing his daily routine?* If a person is putting on his shirt every day, adequate shoulder ROM will probably be maintained. Good hip flexion is required for many transfers. Good hip and knee extension is often needed for successful ambulation.

- *What things would not ordinarily be included in the patient's daily routine?* If a person is W/C dependent and not ambulatory, how will adequate hip extension be maintained? Ankle dorsiflexion is another motion that is frequently lost if the patient is not ambulatory or specifically stretching into this motion. Some have a marked tendency to lose ROM, particularly those with increase in tone. Will ADL be enough to maintain joint motions, or will extra time need to be spent in this area? How will cardiopulmonary endurance be maintained?

- *What are the patient's problem-solving abilities?* If specific problems or potential problem areas were isolated for the patient when discharged, would he be able to attack them in a constructive way? How much guidance will be needed to ensure follow-through?

- *How responsible is the patient?* If he is capable of problem solving, does he use this in his daily routine? Will he take the initiative and direct his care?

- *Family or significant other—what will their role be?* Who will be the primary care giver? How responsible is that person? What is his educational background? How available will he be to carry out a home program?

Having asked these questions, one should now have a fairly good idea of not only *what* needs to be included in the home program but also *how* it should be set up. Not everyone needs an elaborate, well-structured list of exercises. A responsible individual may only need some basic guidelines.

It may be that the home program for some individuals would only include a scheduled time for prone lying to accommodate stretch to the hip flexors, some stretching into dorsiflexion at the ankle, and an allotted time for W/C propulsion to maintain cardiopulmonary endurance. Furthermore, this could feasibly add only an extra five to ten minutes to the patient's daily routine. He would wheel the mile or two home from work (instead of driving) and do his prone lying the first thing in the morning and the last thing in the evening while reading. The extra five to ten minutes would be spent stretching into dorsiflexion at the ankle.

Home programs are an important aspect of any discharge plan; however, successful carryover will be dependent on careful and thorough planning. Home programs should be individualized to each patient, taking into account all the many individual variables including expected levels of independence, discharge plans, and patient life style.

FAMILY TEACHING

The amount of family teaching necessary will vary from patient to patient, depending on many variables: his level of independence, his ability and willingness to direct his care, and the availability and intellectual abilities of family members. However, some guidelines for movement should always be included.

Body mechanics should always be an important consideration, but when a lot of lifting is introduced into one's daily routine (as is often the case for the friend and/or family of an SCI patient), good body mechanics becomes essential. Even if the lift itself is not difficult, the number of times that it is required in a period of time can be stressful if not done correctly.

Body mechanics is nothing more than a way of moving and performing everyday tasks that maintain the normal posture of the back. For the most part, this can be done by directly facing one's tasks and maintaining one's COG within the body's base of support.

The following is a list of some issues to keep in mind during the educational process with the patient and/or significant other:

- *The task should always be assessed first.* How many people are available to assist? In what way will the patient be able to help? Does the patient have special problems to take into account, such as sensitive skin, in which one might need to avoid sliding, or contractures? Early task assessment will provide an opportunity to plan and use the easiest and most efficient method. For instance, the patient and/or significant other may want to transfer closer to the foot of the bed to avoid unnecessary moving once in bed.

- *A wide base of support should be used.* If a family member is assisting with a floor to W/C transfer, his feet should be spread apart rather than being positioned close together.

- *All lifting should be done as close to one's COG as possible* (about waist high). Lifting should not be done with elbows straight. The person or object being lifted should be pulled into the lifter's body *before* lifting.

- *Lower extremity muscles should be used to lift; back muscles should not be used.* The back should be maintained as straight as possible. This may mean starting in a half kneeling or squat position to do a two-man transfer from floor to W/C. The height of a hospital bed should always be adjusted to an appropriate level before any lifting or movement in bed is attempted. The significant other should be reminded to bend his knees as he lowers a W/C down a curb.

- *The lifter should always pivot* (by moving his feet, not twisting his back) *so that he is always facing the patient or object and the direction of movement*. If the patient is being moved to the head of the bed, the mover should face this direction.

- *Energy conservation techniques are frequently helpful*. Instead of lifting the W/C into the car trunk, the use of a ramp could be considered to slide the folded W/C into the trunk. In another instance, a draw sheet could be used under the patient to slide him up and down the bed rather than lifting. When bringing a W/C up the stairs, it is much easier to face the chair away from the stairs, tip it back into a wheelie, and roll the back wheels up the step, one step at a time, than it is to carry it up the stairs. Coming down the stairs, a reverse procedure can be used. If the patient is in the chair, he can assist by controlling the wheel. Using the patient to assist will certainly save energy.

- *Movement is more easily accomplished if the weight can first be shifted off the part being moved*. One method of moving the patient forward within the W/C is to shift his weight (upper trunk and shoulders) to one side and pull the opposite knee forward. This procedure is continued until the patient is appropriately positioned. To position a patient farther back in the W/C, one can use the same method or simply lean the patient forward, taking the weight off the ischium, and pull back at his hips.

ACCESSIBILITY

Even relatively minor disabilities can cause accessibility problems within the environment. People using crutches usually require wider walkways to accommodate the spread of crutches. Any unevenness or debris can be a potential problem in that it is much easier to lose one's balance.

It is not surprising, then, that the person using a W/C as his primary mode of locomotion faces a seemingly unending list of environmental difficulties. Often entrance to a building is prohibited by stairs. Doorways and hallways are not wide enough to allow passage through or turning of a W/C. (Figures 12–1a through 12–1g demonstrate one approach to the problem.) Faucet handles cannot be reached, and storage cabinets are too high. One is only as mobile as his environment allows him to be.

Medical professionals will never be able to solve all these problems, nor should they even expect to. In order for any patient to function independently within his environment, adequate problem-solving skills must be developed. The SCI patient is no exception. The professionals' job is to develop this process and/or to provide the patient with the necessary tools.

The material on the following pages attempts to highlight the process as well as detail some of the tools necessary for this process. Some common W/C dimensions are included as well as some basic considerations regarding maneuvering space in doorways, bathrooms, and bedrooms. Only a few resources have been included in the bibliography, but many exist. Those listed should act as a starting point.

Process of Resolving Accessibility Issues

Establish Needs (Not Wants)

- Determine the level of functional independence.
- Determine the equipment needed to ensure this level of independence.
- Measure dimensions of equipment to be used.
- Evaluate environment (see Assessment Form in Appendix F, Exhibit F–4).
- Refer to available resource material (e.g., Illinois Accessibility Standards) to help clarify and isolate needs (see Bibliography).

Establish What Finances Are Available

Availability may not allow everything to be done at once.

Set Priorities

Major changes should probably not be made right away. Only the bare essentials should be done. After one or two years, the disabled individual usually has a much clearer understanding of what he actually can and cannot do and what his real needs are.

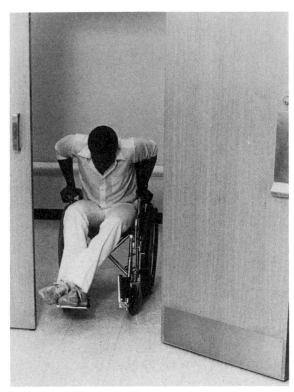

Figure 12–1a Patient is demonstrating how to narrow a W/C to get through narrow door. Step 1: Position chair close to door, lock right brake, and raise left foot pedal.

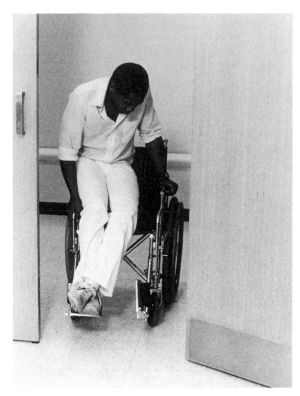

Figure 12–1b Step 2: Lift up to right armrest.

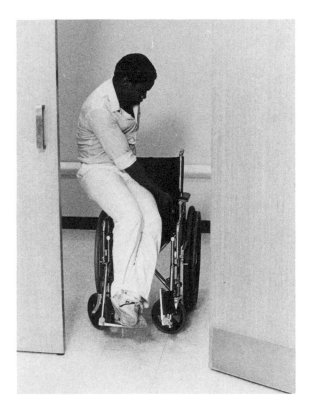

Figure 12–1c Step 3: Pull cushion up and narrow W/C by pulling up on upholstery seat handle. (Note: Many patients also use this sitting position on the armrest to reach for high objects.)

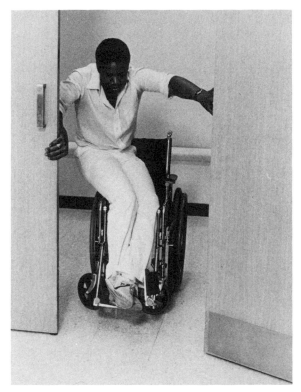

Figure 12–1d Step 4: Unlock brake and pull through the door.

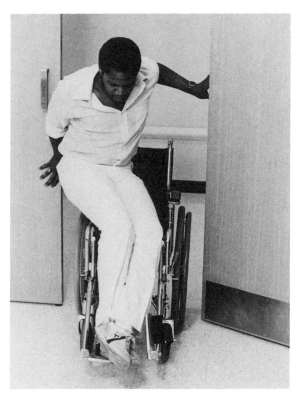

Figure 12–1e

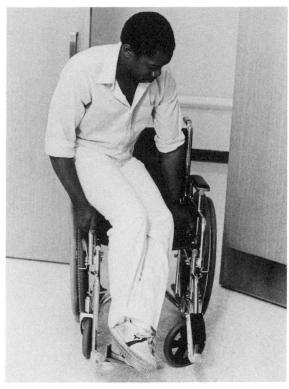

Figure 12–1f Step 5: Push seat rail down, return cushion, and return to seat of W/C.

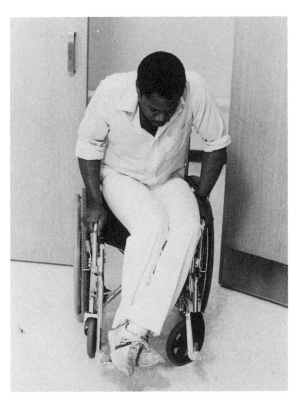

Figure 12–1g

In setting priorities, patients should consider such things as their life style, interests, and family demands. Where will most of their time be spent?

Choose a Vendor to Do the Work

Just like everyone else, the disabled individual should be a comparative consumer. There are companies that specialize in making environments accessible to the disabled; however, any qualified carpenter or construction agency should be able to implement the changes needed once the individual is clear on what should be done; and, this approach is often less expensive.

W/C Dimensions

It would be a tedious, probably impossible, task to include the specific dimensions of all available W/Cs. So only those for a manual adult and an electrically propelled and reclined W/C have been included (Table 12–1). This should serve as a guideline for determination of other W/C dimensions.

TABLE 12–1   Dimensions of Electrically Propelled and Reclined W/Cs*

	Narrow Adult	Standard Adult
Overall width (with trough arms)	27 inches	28 inches
Overall length (with footrests)		
At 90 degrees	48½ inches	
Fully reclined	73½ inches	
Overall height		
With headpiece (will vary, depending on headpiece position)	54 inches	
Without headpiece	42 inches	
Seat height	19 inches	
Turning radius (will vary, depending on how skilled patient is with turning)	6-6½ feet	
Weight	approximately 250 pounds	

*Note: These dimensions may vary a little depending on the W/C and the accessories.

Manual Adult W/C

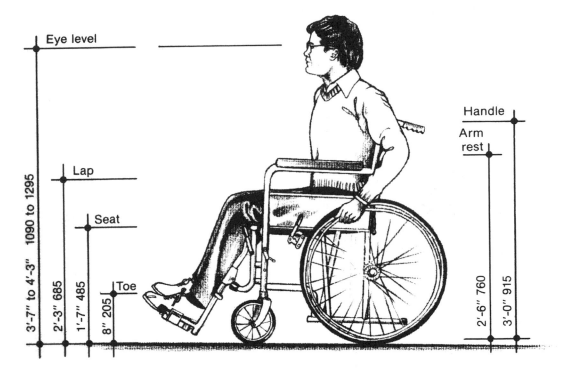

Figure 12–2a Dimensions of a manual, adult sized wheelchair

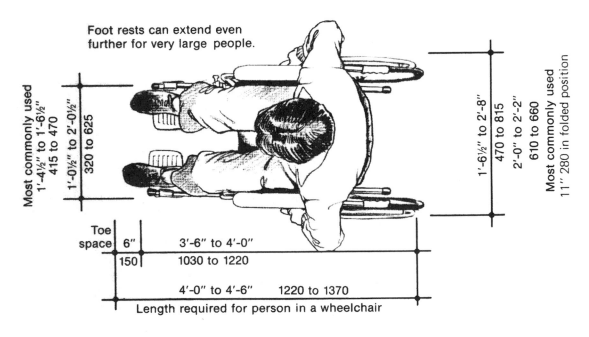

Figure 12–2b

Turning Radius in W/C

The smallest turning radius (Figure 12–3) is achieved by moving one wheel forward while simultaneously moving the other backward to pivot about a point entered just in front of the rear axle.

Reaching Dimensions in W/C

Because of lack of trunk balance, some individuals are unable to lean forward and thus forward reach is restricted (Figures 12–4a and 12–4b).

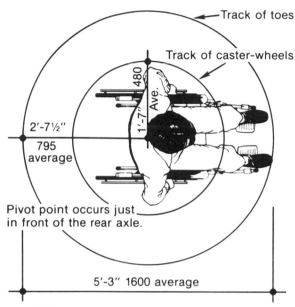

Figure 12–3

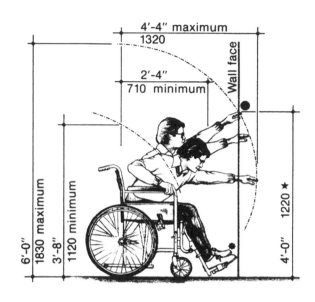

Figure 12–4a Range of forward reach dimension from a wheelchair. (•, Critical point for forward reach at wall condition; ★, highest operable mechanism of any device that can be reached by forward access only; *, toes hitting a wall prevent maximum forward reach from being achieved.)

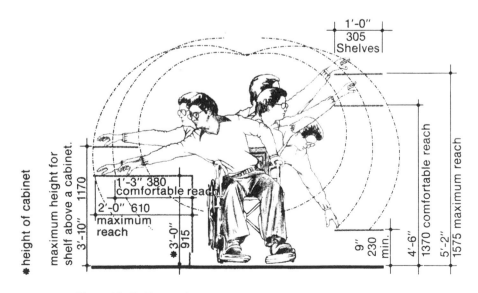

Figure 12–4b Range of reach dimensions on each side of a wheelchair. Narrow shelves and cabinet/worktop are indicated to illustrate furniture constraints.

Maneuvering Space through Doors

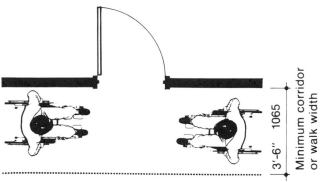

Maneuvering space on push side of door-side approach

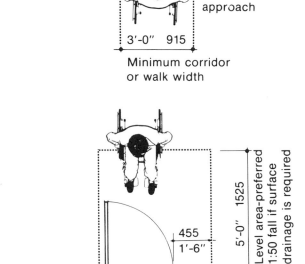

Maneuvering space on push side of door-forward approach

3'-0"   915

Minimum corridor or walk width

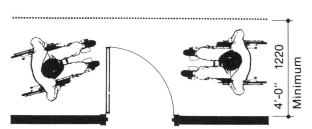

Maneuvering space on pull side of door-side approach

4'-0"   1220   Minimum

Maneuvering space on pull side door-front approach

455
1'-6"

5'-0"   1525   Level area-preferred 1:50 fall if surface drainage is required

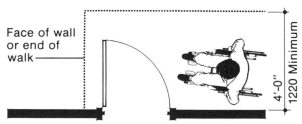

Face of wall or end of walk

1220 Minimum
4'-0"

Doors located at the end of corridors or walks shall have their hinge stiles closest to the corner

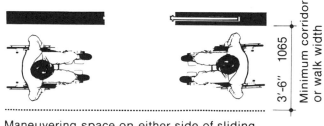

3'-6"   1065   Minimum corridor or walk width

Maneuvering space on either side of sliding door side approach

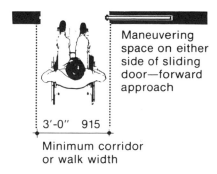

Maneuvering space on either side of sliding door—forward approach

3'-0"   915

Minimum corridor or walk width

Figure 12–5 Maneuvering space at doorways

Maneuvering Space in Bathrooms

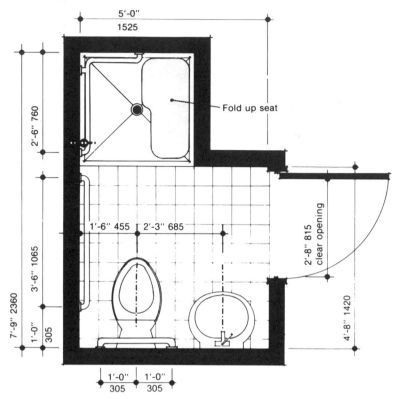

Figure 12–6a Example of minimum size residential bathroom.

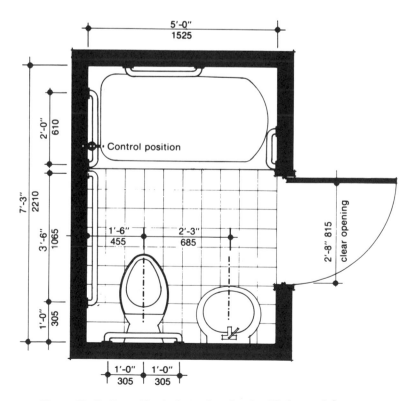

Figure 12–6b Dotted line indicates lengths of wall to have reinforcement to receive grab bars or supports to be supplied by owner/tenant.

Maneuvering Space in Bedrooms

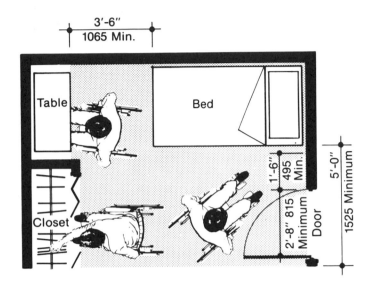

Figure 12–7a Minimum space requirements in accessible bed-rooms: single bed

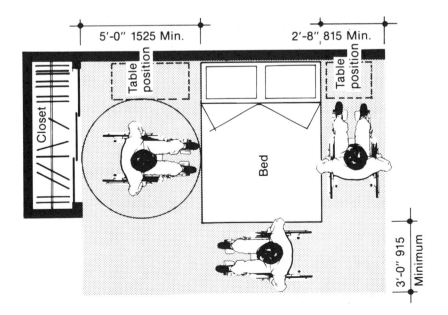

Figure 12–7b Double bed

EQUIPMENT MAINTENANCE

All equipment will last longer if it is well maintained. Some pieces of equipment require more maintenance than others, notably the W/C. Of all equipment prescribed, the W/C probably takes the most stress in day-to-day activities; and yet, with good care, even a W/C can be expected to last up to ten years. Each manufacturer provides a manual with care instructions for each specific W/C. These should be carefully reviewed with each patient.

The average W/C user will probably not do anything but very minor repairs. He should tighten foot pedals, adjust brakes, maintain appropriate tire pressure, and care for the upholstery and metal parts. Unless he really enjoys making repairs, he will probably leave all major repairs to a qualified W/C repair shop. W/Cs should be checked by authorized service personnel every 6 to 12 months.

CONCLUSION

The treatment process for the SCI patient has come to an end—it is time for him to go home. It is hoped that this guide has taught the therapist how to solve problems in treating the SCI patient, in turn enabling the therapist to teach the patient how to solve the problems he will encounter as a disabled person. However, it should be realized that at discharge, most patients still have room for improvement, as they have yet to realize their maximum potentials. From here on, time and practice will be the teachers, enabling patients to improve their proficiency in specific skills. Follow-up visits should be scheduled to monitor progress, as well as to allow patients an opportunity to draw on resources they might not have been able or ready to use in their I/P stay.

In addition, the therapist should recognize that treatment programs for the SCI patient still have much room for growth. Emergency care systems have advanced to the point where they can save the very high-level injuries and yet rehabilitation systems are just beginning to explore how they can impact on these respiratory-dependent patients.

The physical therapy profession has developed much expertise in both the treatment of the orthopedic patient and the neurological patient. However, it has only been recently that therapists have begun to combine their expertise in these two areas. The SCI patients of the 50s are now coming back to P.T. departments with orthopedic problems. Can therapists refine their treatment programs to include techniques that would prevent the development of some of these problems? If therapists place more emphasis on posture and normal joint alignment, would patients complain of less pain in their later years?

The use of FES was only briefly alluded to and yet this is currently an area of intense research. Combining computer technology with electrical stimulation may drastically change the expectations for the SCI patient. Perhaps some day quadriplegic patients will be able to walk, making many of the approaches to ADL discussed in this guide obsolete.

Appendix A
Outcome Summary

C_4	C_5	C_6	C_7	C_8		T_{1-5}	T_{6-8}	T_{9-12}	T_{12}-L_3	L_{4-5}
					Respiration					
X	X	X	X	X	V.C. of at least 30-50% of norm	X	X	X	X	X
X	X	X	X	X	4-5 syllables/breath	X	X	X	X	X
X	X	X	X	X	direct bronchial hygiene	X	X	X	X	X
					Respiration					
	X	X	X	X	V.C. of 40-60% of norm	X	X	X	X	X
	X	X	X	X	6-8 syllables/breath	X	X	X	X	X
	X	X	X	X	assist with bronchial hygiene	X	X	X	X	X
					Respiration					
		X	X	X	V.C. of 60-80% of norm	X	X	X	X	X
		X	X	X	8 syllables/breath	X	X	X	X	X
		?	X	X	independent with bronchial hygiene	X	X	X	X	X
					Respiration					
					V.C. −80% of norm	X	X	X	X	X
					Bed mobility					
X	X	X	X	X	supine → sit with electric bed	X	X	X	X	X
					Bed mobility					
X	X	X	X	X	able to direct	X	X	X	X	X
					Bed mobility					
X	X	X	X	X	patient gives occasional minimal assist	X	X	X	X	X
					Bed mobility					
	X	X	X	X	patient gives moderate assist	X	X	X	X	X

C$_4$	C$_5$	C$_6$	C$_7$	C$_8$		T$_{1-5}$	T$_{6-8}$	T$_{9-12}$	T$_{12}$-L$_3$	L$_{4-5}$
		X	X	X	Bed mobility independent with side rails	X	X	X	X	X
		X	X	X	Bed mobility independent without special equipment	X	X	X	X	X

X	X	X	X	X	Pressure Relief
					    independent with motorized reclining W/C
					      without hand controls
						X	X	X	X	X

X	X	X	X	X	Pressure relief able to direct	X	X	X	X	X

	X	X	X	X	Pressure relief
					    independent with motorized reclining W/C
					      and hand controls
						X	X	X	X	X

	X	X	X	X	Pressure relief assists in manual W/C	X	X	X	X	X
		X	X	X	Pressure relief independent	X	X	X	X	X
		?	X	X	Pressure relief independent including W/C push-ups	X	X	X	X	X
X	X	X	X	X	Transfers able to direct level transfers	X	X	X	X	X
X	X	X	X	X	Transfers able to direct floor to W/C	X	X	X	X	X
	X	X	X	X	Transfers patient gives minimal assist	X	X	X	X	X
		X	X	X	Transfers patient gives moderate assist	X	X	X	X	X
		X	X	X	Transfers independent to and from level surfaces	X	X	X	X	X

			X	X	Transfers
					    patient gives moderate assist with floor to
					      and from W/C
						X	X	X	X	X

			?	?	Transfers independent to and from floor	X	X	X	X	X

X	X	X	X	X	Mobility in W/C
					    independent using motorized W/C without
					      hand controls on level surfaces
						X	X	X	X	X

X	X	X	X	X	Mobility in W/C able to direct	X	X	X	X	X

	X	X	X	X	Mobility in W/C
					    independent using motorized W/C with
					      hand controls on level surfaces
						X	X	X	X	X

C$_4$	C$_5$	C$_6$	C$_7$	C$_8$		T$_{1-5}$	T$_{6-8}$	T$_{9-12}$	T$_{12}$-L$_3$	L$_{4-5}$
	X	X	X	X	Mobility in W/C — independent with manual W/C and oblique projection (200-300 feet forward)	X	X	X	X	X
		X	X	X	Mobility in W/C — independent with manual W/C on level surfaces using vertical projections	X	X	X	X	X
		X	X	X	Mobility in W/C — independent with manual W/C on level surfaces using plastic-coated rims and/or W/C mitts	X	X	X	X	X
			X	X	Mobility in W/C — independent with manual W/C and no special accessories on level surfaces	X	X	X	X	X
			X	X	Mobility in W/C — able to assist on elevations	X	X	X	X	X
					Mobility in W/C — independent in manual W/C on all level surfaces and elevations	X	X	X	X	X
					Ambulation — independent with bilateral KAFO in "P" bars	?	X	X	X	X
					Ambulation — supervision with bilateral KAFO and walker	?	X	X	X	X
					Ambulation — independent with bilateral KAFO and walker			?	X	X
					Ambulation — independent with bilateral KAFO and Lofstands			X	X	X
					Ambulates using bilateral KAFO and Lofstands with supervision on elevations and rough terrain			X	X	X
					Ambulation — independent with bilateral KAFO and Lofstands on all surfaces				X	X
					Ambulation — independent with bilateral AFO with crutches or canes					X
		X	X	X	Self-ROM — able to assist	X	X	X	X	X
			X	X	Self-ROM — independent	X	X	X	X	X

Common Substitutions in Manual Muscle Testing*

UPPER EXTREMITIES AND SCAPULA

Upper Trapezius

- Levator scapulae can substitute; however get scapular elevation and adduction of the medial border of scapula.

Middle Trapezius

- Rhomboids can substitute; however get scapular adduction and medial-interior rotation of the inferior angle of scapula.
- Levator scapula can possibly substitute; it produces scapular elevation and adduction of the medial border scapula.

Rhomboids

- Middle trapezius can substitute, giving pure adduction of medial border scapula.
- Patient can lift hand off buttock using the shoulder extensors (posterior deltoid, teres major, latissimus dorsi and long head triceps).

- Patient can also lift hand off buttock by tipping the scapula forward using the pectorals, especially pectoralis minor with coracobrachialis.

Serratus Anterior

- Pectoralis minor and coracobrachialis can substitute by tipping scapula forward.
- Scapula should not wing off the chest/thoracic wall as the patient assumes the prone-on-elbows position.

Biceps

- Brachioradialis can substitute where elbow flexion occurs in the mid position of pronation and supination; the patient cannot bend the elbow in full supination (remember the main action of biceps is supination).

Pectoralis Major

- In terms of the adduction/internal rotation components of this muscle's activity, the patient can substitute with the long head of biceps, coracobrachialis, and anterior deltoid, possibly latissimus dorsi.
- Remember the segmental innervation for the clavicular components of pectoralis major is C5-6 while the segmental innervation of the sternal

---

*All the information in this appendix was developed by Ann Charness, M.S., P.T., a current staff member, as part of her teaching materials used when she was on the P.T. faculty at the University of Minnesota.

components of pectoralis major is C7-8–T1 (possibly a small amount of C6).

- If the patient is prone on elbows and is shifting weight side to side to shift weight onto the right elbow and forearm, patient can use left middle deltoid to abduct and shift away from the left then to use right long head biceps and coracobrachialis for the final shift to the right.

Triceps

- Straightening the elbow with the arm free in space, the patient will use the external rotators of the shoulder (supraspinatus, infraspinatus, teres minor) to place the arm in a position where gravity will straighten the elbow, which is kept extended by a bony locking of the olecranon process and the humerus; brachioradialis can help.
- While straightening the elbow with the patient's weight bearing on the arm, the patient will use some external rotation of the shoulder coupled with gravity; however, some of the final locking of the elbow in extension is done by the pectoralis major, the long head of biceps, and the coracobrachialis.

Deltoid

- Paralysis of the middle fibers is compensated for by the long head of biceps, long head of triceps, clavicular pectoralis, major external rotators of shoulder, and serratus anterior.

Shoulder External Rotators

- Patient can substitute by depressing shoulder so that gravity can rotate the shoulder.
- Patient will also try to use the supinators of the forearm and the extensors of the wrist to help rotate wrist and arm with gravity.

Supinator

- Biceps, as well as shoulder external rotators, brachioradialis, and wrist extensors can substitute.

Shoulder Internal Rotators

- Pectoralis minor and coracobrachialis can substitute by tipping shoulder forward so gravity can rotate shoulder internally.

- Patient can also substitute with pronators, wrist flexors, and brachioradialis.

Pronators

- Patient can substitute with shoulder internal rotators and brachioradialis.

Wrist Extensors

- Patient can substitute by externally rotating shoulder so that gravity can extend the wrist.
- Patient can substitute by supinating the forearm so that gravity can extend the wrist.
- Patient can substitute with any of the long finger extensors.

Wrist Flexors

- Patient can substitute by internally rotating shoulder so that gravity can flex the wrist.
- Patient can substitute by pronating the forearm so that gravity can flex the wrist.

Latissimus Dorsi

- Patient can substitute with teres major, post deltoid, lower trapezius, and possible long head of triceps.

Long Finger Flexors

- Be aware of the tenedesis effect whereby wrist extension produces passive tension on the long finger flexors; some finger flexion especially at the interphalangeal joints can occur.

Long Finger Extensors

- Be aware of the tenedesis effect whereby wrist flexion produces passive tension on the long finger extensors; some finger extension especially at the interphalangeal joints can occur.

TRUNK

Abdominals (Upper)

- Patient can substitute with head and neck flexors, pectoralis major and minor, and serratus anterior.

Obliques

- Patient can substitute with latissimus dorsi so long as the hands are fixed on the treatment surface.

Quadrantus Lumborum

- Patient can substitute with latissimus dorsi as above.

LOWER EXTREMITIES

Hip Flexors

- Patient can substitute with the lower abdominals, which tilt the pelvis backward and cause the leg to swing forward with momentum.
- Patient can substitute with lower obliques, which rotate the pelvis forward, causing the leg to swing forward.
- Know that hip adductors can flex hip.
- Know that latissimus dorsi can cause some flexion and abduction of the hip as the patient hikes his pelvis.

Hip Extensors

- Patient can substitute with the lower back extensor muscles, which tilt the pelvis forward and cause the leg to swing backward with momentum.
- Realize that you may think you feel some hip extensors simply as the patient maximally contracts the hip flexors. As he lets go and relaxes, the leg will move back on rebound or recoil.
- Patient can substitute with the longitudinal fibers of adductor magnus.
- Patient can substitute with quadratus lumborum.

Hip Abductors

- Patient can substitute for gluteus medius and minimus using either latissimus dorsi or the obliques to hike the pelvis.
- Patient can substitute with sartorius, which will flex.
- Patient can abduct the hip as well with tensor fascia lata.

Hip Adductors

- Patient can substitute using lower abdominal muscles.
- Patient can substitute with some of the hip flexors.
- Patient can substitute using lower abdominals to rotate the pelvis forward, allowing gravity to adduct the leg.

Hip Internal Rotators

- Patient can substitute using lower abdominal muscles to rotate the pelvis forward so gravity internally rotates the leg.

Hip External Rotators

- Patient can substitute using lower back extensors to rotate the pelvis backward so gravity externally rotates the leg.

Knee Flexors

- Patient can substitute for semimembranosus and semitendinosus using sartorius and gracilis.
- Patient can substitute with the rebound phenomenon from the quadriceps.

Quadriceps

- Patient can substitute in sitting position simply by leaning the trunk backward, thus initiating a swinging motion of the legs upward.
- Patient can substitute in lying position by using adductor magnus to extend the hip; if the knee is flexed it will also straighten out.

Foot Inversion

- Patient can substitute by rotating the hips inward and with the medial gastrocnemius.

Foot Eversion

- Patient can substitute by rotating the hip outward and with the lateral gastrocnemius.

Autonomic Hyperreflexia and Ectopic Bone

There are two medical conditions that are important to mention in this guide: autonomic hyperreflexia and ectopic bone.

AUTONOMIC HYPERREFLEXIA

All therapists working with SCI patients should be familiar with the causes and symptoms of hyperreflexia and prepared to deal immediately with this emergency situation. Failure to respond immediately could result in elevated blood pressure sufficient to produce a cerebral vascular accident. This condition can occur in any patient with a lesion above the T5 level. It is generally caused by a distended bladder or distended rectum (usually by feces) or by other stimuli about the sacral innervated areas associated with urological procedures in catheterization or bladder irrigation.

The symptoms are pounding headache, hypertension, sweating above the level of the SCI, piloerection, slow pulse, and nasal obstruction. All symptoms are aggravated by supine positioning.

If the spine is stable, position the patient in sitting immediately to create postural hypotension or decreased blood pressure, check the catheter and tubing for plugging or kinking. Empty legbag if it is full (never allow legbag to become full). If symptoms persist, follow the facility's protocol for obtaining immediate medical and/or nursing attention.

ECTOPIC BONE

Ectopic bone or hypertrophic bone appears to occur frequently in the SCI population. It seems to occur predominantly in males and unilaterally or bilaterally in the hips. Other joints may be affected as well. The suggested precaution is an aggressive stretching exercise for ROM. Physicians should be consulted. Although maintaining range is essential for functional activity and W/C positioning, it is important never to attempt forward pressure stretching from the trunk onto legs (as in long sitting), which could result in femoral fractures. This is strongly discouraged in any instance owing to possibilities of femoral fractures, lumbar fractures, or overstretching low back musculature needed for sitting balance.

As already indicated, the patient with ectopic bone will present many unique problems in therapy associated with W/C positioning and pressure distribution and with short sitting balance unsupported by upper extremities and some transfers.

Functional Electrical Stimulation*

TREATMENT GOALS

- muscle strengthening
- ROM
- increase sensory awareness
- muscle facilitation
- orthotic substitution
- transient spasticity management
- decrease venous stasis

CONTRAINDICATIONS

- cardiac—exercise caution; monitor cardiac status before, during, and after (i.e., pulse, blood pressure, electrocardiogram, if available); over carotid sinus; never stimulate over the carotid sinus; cardiac pacemakers. Never stimulate patients who have pacemakers.
- skin—no stimulation over skin lesions; use caution with fragile skin; beware of hypersensitivity to gel and tape.

---

*All information in this appendix was developed by Jane Sullivan, P.T., a current staff member, as an outline for a series of staff inservices. Ms. Sullivan is now actively involved in research on this subject.

- orthopedic—do not stimulate in orthopedically unstable areas unless immobilized.

INTERFERING FACTORS

- obesity. It will be necessary to increase the amplitude to get current through adipose tissue; this may result in a noxious stimuli.
- peripheral neuropathy. Success is limited with partially innervated muscle. A longer pulse duration (possibly DC stimulation) may be required. The results may be better proximal versus distal.

GENERAL PRINCIPLES

1. Skin Preparation:
   a. The skin area must be cleaned (mild soap or alcohol can be used).
   b. The area can be shaved if excessive hair is present.
2. Generous amounts of gel should be used to cover the entire electrode to increase transmission and avoid "burning" sensations.
   a. Pre-gelled, self-adhesive electrodes are available as well as gel "pads," such as karaya pads.
   b. The electrodes should be well secured with tape.
   c. It is generally best to secure the distal electrode first and probe for the most effective response with the proximal electrode (usually over the

motor point). When looking for the most effective placement of electrodes, the constant stimulation button can be used to avoid waiting for a complete cycle at each location.

3. The electrodes may be left in place for up to one week, provided they remain secure.
   a. Use of tape patches is recommended for more than one treatment session.
   b. If the patient complains of a burning sensation, check for loosening of the electrodes or inadequate gel.

4. Discomfort from the stimulator may be an early limiting factor. It may require up to a week for the patient to tolerate the necessary level of stimulation. Electric stimulation is a new sensory experience for most patients; however, if good patient-therapist rapport is established, patients can learn to tolerate the sensation. Stimulation beyond the range of comfortable sensation should be avoided, especially during the early stages of treatment.

5. Parameters:
   a. Amplitude (generally measured in milliamperes) is determined by individual tolerance and motor response. With increasing amplitude, more and deeper fibers are stimulated.
   b. Frequency—rate, pulses/second, or hertz (Hz). Contractions will be "jerky" with lower frequencies (below approximately 20 Hz). At higher frequencies the fatigue factor must be considered.
   c. Surge or ramp time—the time it takes the current to go from zero to maximum. If no spasticity is present, the ramp time is determined by patient comfort and desired motor response. If spasticity is a factor, the ramp time should be long. When working with spasticity and using a long ramp, the on-time must exceed the ramp time enough to provide adequate time for a maximal contraction (i.e., if the ramp time is 8 seconds the on-time should be 12 to 15 seconds). When using accessories (e.g., heel switch), the desired response may be quick; therefore a fast ramp time should be used.
   d. Fall time—the time it takes the current to go from maximum to zero; may be a factor with spastic muscles
   e. On-off time ("duty cycle")—a good starting point is 1:4 or 1:5, stimulation:rest. Gradually build the patient's tolerance as endurance increases. The small light on the outside of the unit indicates the on-off cycle and serves as a

good visual feedback to patients. The patient should be encouraged to use this feedback if appropriate.

   Note: Total amount of stimulation can be increased as fatigue resistance increases. This can be done by increasing the treatment time (e.g., from 15 minutes twice daily to 30 minutes), and increasing the ratio of stimulation to rest (e.g., 1:4 to 1:3, 1:2, 1:1, 2:1 and so on).

6. Accessories:
   a. Heel switch—can provide stimulation when weight is taken off the heel; therefore stimulation ends at heel strike. It can then be used to stimulate during the swing phase of gait. Stimulation can also be provided when weight is put on the heel to stimulate during stance phase.
   b. Trigger switch—provides stimulation "at the touch of a button" and can be controlled by patient or therapist

SPASTICITY MANAGEMENT

Guidelines

Usually 20 to 30 minutes, administered immediately before another treatment. (May need to increase time with increased spasticity.) Stimulation is of the antagonist. This is thought to work because of reciprocal inhibition. It is typically used before facilitation or functional training. The decrease in spasticity is temporary. Frequently there is longer carryover after multiple sessions.

Examples

- Stimulate quadriceps to decrease hamstring tone before gait or transfer training
- Stimulate anterior tibialis and/or foot evertors to decrease plantarflexor tone before upright activities.

FACILITATION/SENSORY AWARENESS

Stimulation of one or two muscles can be done during a functional activity

Theories

- Repetitive stimulation increases the excitability of the alpha motor neuron pool.

- Increased sensory motor awareness is developed through stimulation.

This treatment needs the patient's cooperation. It is not passive stimulation. It works well with rhythmic activities and can also be good with apraxics patients.

Examples

- weight-shifting activities. Any muscle used during weight bearing can be stimulated cyclically or with a heel switch during weight shifting activities (i.e., hip extensors, hip abductors, quads). Two muscles may be stimulated simultaneously.
- table-top activities. Stimulate one or two muscles during reaching or prehension activities; use trigger switch.

DECREASE VENOUS STASIS

Venous stasis is decreased by activating the "muscle pump" mechanism at or distal to the area.

ROM

ROM can be maintained or stimulation can be used for correction of contractures. The muscles are stimulated through the full available range. The patient is positioned so gravity can assist in stretching muscles. For example, when stretching hip flexors by stimulating hip extensors, the most advantageous position would be supine.

A more extensive program is needed at a joint where muscle imbalance exists (e.g., gastrocnemius/anterior compartment or quadriceps/hamstrings).

Stimulation can be used in conjunction with splinting or casting (e.g., stimulation of triceps during drop-out casting for elbow extension).

The mechanics and possible pathology of the joint and surrounding structures must always be considered before undertaking a vigorous stimulation program.

STRENGTHENING PROGRAMS

Strengthening programs is an area of a great deal of controversy with respect to stimulation. In evaluating FES as an adjunct in a strengthening program, consider the following:

- Stimulation may affect motor relearning or muscle reeducation.

- When spasticity is present, stimulation may be effective in decreasing tone, thereby allowing a weak agonist to work more effectively, the end result being increased strength in the agonist.
- Several studies have demonstrated increasing fatigue resistance through stimulation. This individual muscle fatigue resistance may be viewed as a component of "strength."

When generalized weakness is present, it is generally best to select the muscle most significant for function or the most proximal muscle and start there. Remember that one or two muscles may be stimulated, unilaterally or bilaterally, simultaneously or reciprocally, cyclically (rhythmically), or during a functional activity. Trigger switches can be used to initiate the motion and allow the patient to complete it actively or, conversely, to complete the motion once the patient has completed a portion (e.g., terminal knee extension).

Upgrading programs is done in much the same way as with "conventional" strengthening programs. The "degree of difficulty" of only one variable should be increased at a time. Variables are total treatment time/ day, ratio of stimulation to rest, plane of motion (gravity eliminated versus against gravity), and external resistance.

ORTHOTIC SUBSTITUTION

FES may be used as a definitive orthotic device or in conjunction with an orthosis.

Gait Activities

FES can be used during gait to stimulate muscles during swing or stance phase, using accessories (i.e., heel switch or trigger switch). Optimal electrode placement for the muscle to be stimulated must first be determined.

Swing Phase

The trigger or heel switch may be used. The heel switch can provide stimulation when weight is taken off the heel. Stimulation ends at heel strike. Muscles that may be stimulated (two muscles may be stimulated simultaneously) are anterior tibialis, evertors, hamstrings, hip abductors, and hip flexors.

Stance Phase

Either the trigger or heel switch is used. Muscles that may be stimulated (two muscles may be stimulated simultaneously) are quadriceps, hip abductors, hip adductors, and hip extensors.

Examples

- "buckling" knee—weak quadriceps. Use cyclic stimulation or accessories with weight shifting or during gait, frequently both weak hip extensors and quadriceps are a problem and can be stimulated simultaneously.

- "scissoring" in gait. Stimulate abductors with cyclic stimulation or with the heel switch during gait.

- ankle weakness. Facilitation and strengthening can be done to anterior tibialis and/or evertors with cyclic stimulation or with the heel switch during gait.

Class Exercise Programs*

The following is a broad outline of class exercise programs currently being held in the Physical Therapy Department of the Rehabilitation Institute of Chicago. Depending on the needs of the population being treated at any given time, the programs are altered to meet those needs. Class exercise programs in this respect do not differ from any other physical therapy treatment programs. A class exercise program augments and achieves the same goals as a patient's individual treatment program.

SLING CLASS

Goals

- to maximize muscle strength of upper and lower extremities

Activities

- gravity eliminated───▶gravity eliminated–resisted

- individualized pace and intensity
- individualized target muscle groups

Population

- Patients with upper and/or lower extremity musculature of below fair muscle grades (e.g., those with SCI, multiple sclerosis, Guillain-Barré syndrome, cerebral vascular accident, and head injury)

Equipment

- raised mats or plinths and pillows
- sling suspension overhead grid
- canvas slings
- "S" hooks
- sling ropes with wooden cleats
- springs

Staff

- one PT
- one PT aide (additional aides available for transfers)

---

*All information in this appendix was developed by a staff member, Jane Sullivan, P.T., as a special project for designing a class tutorial which allows other therapists/facilities to learn this approach to patient care.

BEGINNING UPPER EXTREMITY CLASS

Goals

- maximize upper extremity strength
- maximize neck strength
- maximize endurance
- maximize cardiorespiratory fitness
- reinforce bed mobility and sitting balance as taught by primary therapist

Activities

- upper extremity and neck exercises
- active assistive ────→ active ────→ resistive (as possible)
- variety of concentric, eccentric, and isometric exercises
- variety of breathing exercises
- speed and endurance exercises
- warm up and cool down exercises
- sitting balance and mat mobility activities

Population

- patients with significant weakness or loss of function in the upper extremities (e.g., C4 and C5 quadriplegics, those with Guillain-Barré syndrome)

Equipment

- cuff weights
- floor mats and pillows
- elbow splints helpful
- optional: bean bag chairs, balloons, blow bubbles

Staff

- one PT
- one PT aide (approximately eight PT aides for W/C to floor transfers)
- volunteers as possible (optimally one volunteer or staff member per patient)

INTERMEDIATE UPPER EXTREMITY CLASS

Goals

- maximize upper extremity strength
- maximize neck strength
- maximize endurance
- maximize cardiorespiratory fitness
- reinforce bed mobility and sitting balance as taught by primary therapist

Activities

- active assistive ────→ active ────→ resistive exercise
- variety of concentric, eccentric, and isometric exercises
- variety of breathing exercises
- warm up and cool down exercises
- sitting balance activities

Population

- patients with significant weakness or loss of function in the upper extremities (e.g., C5, C6, C7 quadriplegics, those with Guillain-Barré syndrome or multiple sclerosis)

Equipment

- cuff weights
- floor mats and pillows
- optional: bean bag chairs, balls, balloons, game/sport equipment

Staff

- one PT
- one PT aide
- volunteers as possible (approximately eight aides available for W/C to floor transfers)

ADVANCED UPPER EXTREMITY CLASS

Goals

- maximize upper extremity strength
- maximize neck and trunk strength
- maximize endurance
- maximize cardiorespiratory fitness
- reinforce bed mobility and sitting balance as taught by primary therapist

Activities

- active progressing to resistive exercises
- variety of concentric, eccentric, and isometric exercises
- incorporated with breathing exercises
- speed exercises
- endurance exercises
- warm up stretches
- cool down exercises
- mobility activities (rolling, sitting, W/C to floor transfers)
- breathing activities
- sport/game activities (e.g., volleyball, tetherball, basketball, bowling)

Population

- patients with intact but weak upper extremity musculature (e.g., paraplegics, low level quadriplegics, amputees, those with multiple sclerosis or Guillain-Barré syndrome)

Equipment

- weights (cuff and dumbbell)
- floor mats and pillows
- sport/game equipment

Staff

- one PT
- one PT aide (approximately eight aides for transfers)

Miscellaneous

- two sessions (one in morning, one in afternoon), with patients enrolled in one or the other

LOWER EXTREMITY STRENGTHENING CLASS

Goals

- maximize lower extremity strength
- maximize trunk strength
- maximize endurance
- reinforce bed mobility skills and developmental activities as taught by the primary therapist

Activities (see Exhibit E–1) Lower Extremity and Trunk Strengthening

- active assistive———active———resistive exercise
- variety of concentric, eccentric, and isometric exercises
- speed and endurance exercises
- warm up and cool down exercises
- developmental activities

Population

- patients with lower extremity weakness (generally fair or above) (e.g., incomplete or low level SCI, multiple sclerosis, Guillain-Barré, amputees, higher level cerebral vascular accident and head injured)

Equipment

- cuff weights
- floor mats and pillows
- optional: bean bags, game equipment (rings, balls, balloons, dental dam)

Staff

- one PT
- one PT aide (additional aides available for transfers as needed)

Exhibit E–1 Characteristics of Strengthening Class

A. Warm Up Period
   1. Stretching
   2. Cardiovascular warm up
   3. Lower resistance and repetitions of exercises
B. Vigorous Activity
   1. Varied types of *movements*
      a. Isolated joint movements
      b. Multiple muscle movements (e.g., PNF diagonals)
   2. Varied types of Muscle *Contractions*
      a. Eccentric
      b. Concentric
      c. Isometric
   3. Exercises for power: high resistance/low repetition
   4. Exercises for endurance: high repetition/low resistance
   5. Exercises for speed: low resistance/high speed
   6. Exercises for coordination: low resistance/low progressing to higher speed
   7. Resisted functional activities (e.g., rolling/push-ups with weights or manual resistance)
   8. Repetitive function activities (e.g., repetitive practice of supine ←→ sitting)
   9. Exercises combined with specific breathing patterns
C. Cool Down Period
   1. Stretching
   2. Low resistance/low repetition exercises
   3. Relaxation

Progress can be documented and evaluated by initial evaluation of the following parameters:

- pre/post exercise heart rate
- pre/post exercise respiratory rate
- repetitions of particular exercises
- resistance tolerated with particular exercises
- rest periods required/exercise period
- vital capacity

Records of these measures can be kept by the class therapist, primary therapist, or patient.

Patients may be encouraged to continue upgrading their baseline measurements or work toward a predetermined goal (e.g., 75 percent of predicted normal vital capacity, 20 percent increase over resting heart rate in one exercise class, and so on).

Exhibit E–2 Prerequisites and Specific Goals for Quadriplegic W/C Class

Prerequisites

- beginning propulsion of manual W/C
- introduction to W/C skills on checklist

Specific Goals

1. Increased endurance (increased number of laps/time) in W/C propulsion
2. Increased speed in propulsion (decreased time for one lap)
3. Increased ability to manage W/C parts; if not independent in management, patient is able to instruct others
   a. Armrests
   b. Footplates
   c. Brakes
   d. Ramp retarders
4. Ability to manage wheelchair outdoors within limits of spinal cord lesion; if not independent, patient has ability to instruct another
   a. Level sidewalks
   b. Slanted sidewalks
   c. Rough terrain
   d. Ramps 1:10, 1:5
   e. Curbs: one to six inches
5. Ability to maneuver W/C on the level: forward, backward, and turns
6. Ability to move on carpeting (may be limited with lesion level)
7. Ability to relieve pressure independently or with spotting.
   a. Leaning forward
   b. Sideways
   c. Push ups
8. Ability to fall safely from W/C and ability to direct return to W/C.
9. Ability to direct W/C repair and prevention of problems
   a. Change a tire
   b. Tighten brakes
   c. Adjust footplates
10. Daily class activities:
   a. Monday—timing of laps, endurance activities and individual skills
   b. Tuesday—go outdoors if possible
   c. Thursday—obstacle course
   d. Friday—group games
11. Individual therapist responsibilities
   a. Fill out patient's initial mobility level on checklist
   b. Check expected level of achievement with (*) on checklist; class therapist will fill out progress

QUADRIPLEGIC W/C CLASS

Goals

- maximize independence (and/or ability to direct care) in W/C mobility and management (see Exhibit E–2)
- maximize cardiovascular fitness
- maximize endurance
- patient exposure to game/sport activities

Activities

- endurance runs
- obstacle courses
- W/C part management practice
- pressure relief methods

- W/C mobility on a variety of surfaces and elevations as possible
- *note:* this class is frequently held outdoors to facilitate accomplishment of mobility goals.

Population

- patients with mid- and low-level quadriplegia, multiple sclerosis, and Guillain-Barré syndrome

Equipment

- floor mats
- materials for obstacle course
- sport/game equipment
- ramps

Staff

- one PT
- one PT aide
- volunteers as possible (optimally one volunteer or staff member per patient)

ADVANCED W/C CLASS

Goals

- maximize independence in W/C mobility skills
- maximize independence in W/C management/maintenance skills
- maximize cardiovascular fitness
- maximize endurance
- patient exposure to game/sport activities

Activities

- W/C exercises
- endurance runs
- obstacle courses
- W/C maintenance activities
- wheelies and curb jumping (see Exhibit E–3)
- pressure relief
- W/C to floor transfers
- W/C mobility on a variety of surfaces
- exposure to sports activities
- *note:* this class is frequently held outdoors to facilitate accomplishment of mobility goals.

Exhibit E–3 Advanced W/C Skills Class Worksheet

	Date Completed
A. Wheelie	
Maintain balance in wheelie	_____
Move 10 feet forward in wheelie	_____
Turn in wheelie	_____
B. Curbs	
1. Four inches or less (low curb)	
a. Front casters-back wheels	_____
b. Running start	_____
2. Four inches or more (high curb)	
a. Stationary	_____
b. Running start	_____
3. Back down	_____
4. Forward-down curb in wheelie	_____
C. Ramps	
1. 1:10	
a. Ascend	_____
b. Descend	_____
c. Descend in wheelie	_____
2. 1.5	
a. Ascend	_____
b. Descend	_____
c. Descend in wheelie	_____
D. Transfers	
1. W/C to and from floor with steps	_____
2. W/C to and from floor: out	_____
3. W/C to and from floor: in	_____
E. Outdoor Skills	
1. Level sidewalks	_____
2. Unlevel sidewalks	_____
3. Rough terrain	_____
a. Curbs	_____
b. Ramps	_____
F. Falling Techniques	_____
G. Up stairs with W/C (optional)	_____
H. In and out of car with W/C (optional)	_____
I. W/C parts management	
1. Fix brakes	_____
2. Adjust footrests	_____
3. Tighten spokes	_____

Population

- patients with potential for partial or total independence in outdoor wheelchair skills (e.g., paraplegics or low-level quadriplegics, amputees, those with multiple sclerosis)

Equipment

- floor mat(s)
- curbs

- ramps
- tools
- sport/game equipment

Staff

- one PT
- one PT aide
- volunteers as available (optimally one volunteer or staff member per patient)

ADVANCED GAIT CLASS

Goals

- maximize quality and independence in level surface gait activities
- maximize quality and independence in advanced gait activities
- maximize endurance
- reinforce independence in transfer techniques as taught by primary therapist

Activities

- warm up sitting or standing activities
- standing activities (supported or unsupported) (e.g., weight shift, balance, foot placement)
- gait activities (with assistive device if needed) including all directions, all surfaces, elevations, all speeds, distance, and obstacles
- game/sport activities
- *note:* This class frequently meets outside to facilitate accomplishment of goals.

Population

- patients who require minimal assistance or less to ambulate (e.g., those with cerebral vascular accidents, head injuries, low level or incomplete SCI, multiple sclerosis, or Guillain-Barré syndrome and amputees)

Equipment

- variety of assistive devices
- temporary orthoses and lifts
- gait belts

- straight-backed chairs
- sport/game equipment

Staff

- one PT
- one PT aide
- volunteers as available (optimally one volunteer or staff member per patient)

SPECIAL CONSIDERATIONS

Examples of special considerations in class management are presented in Exhibit E–4 using the criteria established by the Rehabilitation Institute of Chicago.

Exhibit E–4 Special Considerations in Class Management at the Rehabilitation Institute of Chicago

1. No patient will be admitted to class with a specific pulse or blood pressure limit set by the physician. Class therapists are not able to individually routinely monitor patients but will do so in the case of patient distress. Patients may be admitted if the physician has indicated cardiac precautions, without a specific pulse or blood pressure limit.
2. Patients who require suctioning may be admitted provided they are accompanied by a private duty nurse who can suction them. The class therapist cannot suction patients while conducting class.
3. Blind and/or deaf patients will be admitted provided they are able to join in the class activity and follow directions of the class therapist. *Note:* In some classes, staff and/or volunteer help is frequently available on a 1:1 (patient:staff) basis. The need for this assistance should be discussed with the class therapist and/or class supervisor.
4. Patients on wound and skin isolation may attend class provided the infected area is covered with a dressing and clothing.
5. Patients on secretion isolation may not attend class unless a private duty nurse is available to handle their secretions with sterile technique.
6. Patients with urinary tract infections and on excretion isolation may attend class. Leg bag emptying procedure is outlined in the *Infection Control Manual*. Attempts will be made to empty leg bags before or after class if necessary.
7. Patients demonstrating combative, abusive, or disruptive behavior will be discontinued from the class program at the discretion of the class therapist and class supervisor.
8. Patients on oxygen therapy will be admitted to classes that occur in one area and do not require extensive movement (e.g., strengthening classes). They will not be admitted to mobility oriented classes (W/C, gait) unless accompanied by someone who can push oxygen cylinder.
9. When class size becomes unmanageable, patients with poor attendance may be discontinued at the discretion of the class therapist and supervisor.
10. Patients late for class may be turned away at the discretion of the class therapist.

GUIDELINES FOR DEVELOPING AND EVALUATING CLASS PROGRAMS

Punctuality

- starting and ending on time

Safety

- spacing of patients
- positioning of patients
- supervision of transfers
- removal of obstacles so that area is cleared and safe for class activities
- instruction of supportive staff in safety factors
- safe use of equipment
- appropriateness of weights and other equipment for patients
- physical coverage of class at all times
- visual coverage of class at all times
- adequate guarding of patients
- handling of patients
- awareness of individual precautions

Programs

- preparation of program, including equipment to be used
- selection of exercises appropriate to population
- combination of exercises to achieve goals and not overload one aspect
- sequencing of activities (e.g., warm up activity, work, wind down)
- variety of program's intensity
- appropriate use of games or sports to reach therapy goals
- use of class setting to instruct patients

Delivery

- posture and body language
- clarity of speech
- loudness of voice
- pace of speech
- appropriateness of tone
- atmosphere created
- promotion of motivation
- choice of words for instruction
- leadership and control of class

Demonstration

- accurate
- precise
- visible to all
- repeated when necessary

Pacing of Class

- pacing of the class as a whole
- speed of individual exercises/activities
- appropriateness of the above two factors to the population
- smooth and uninterrupted transition from one activity/exercise to the next

Patient Supervision

- observation of patient's performance
- appropriate correction and/or instruction
- offers constructive feedback

Supervision and Utilization of Personnel

- direction of personnel to assist in providing continuity to the class
- adequate use of personnel
- adequate instruction both before and during class session, including such items as feedback to volunteers as to their performance, correction of their dress if inappropriate or unsafe (e.g., footwear)

Initiative

- creativity of programs
- variety of exercises/activities
- variety of equipment used
- use of resource material and people

KEY TO THE PHYSICAL THERAPY ADL FORM (EXHIBIT F–2)

Usage

The ADL form is to be completed on all patients with goals in ADL training and on a *recheck* evaluation when an ADL form has been completed previously.

Purpose

The form is designed to determine a patient's *highest level of independence*. If a more advanced skill requiring more assistance can be performed by a patient, this should be included in the PT progress notes. *Example:* Patient walks independently with a pick-up walker, but training was just begun with two standard canes. The ADL form should reflect his highest level of independent walking, therefore the walker. However, mention of the two standard canes should be made in the PT progress notes.

Source of Data

The evaluation is to be a *test by performance for any grade above (2) dependent*. Information must not be recorded on the basis of patient/family testimony.

Frequency of Testing

Testing should be performed at time of admission, at discharge, and at least one time during the interim period. (Exceptions would include short admissions when time does not allow for interim testing). At discharge, note in the last column with an (x) those skills the family has demonstrated competency in performing, assisting, or supervising.

Grading Key

1. *Not tested.* For this Grade write the abbreviation N.T. in the box under Column 1. Not tested is to be used in the following situations:

   - Patient refuses the test
   - Inclement weather
   - Outpatient recheck (state specific goal of recheck or time)

   State the reason for *not* testing an item on the lines below the category. If an item is contraindicated at this time, patient is *dependent* in performing it and should be marked Grade 2. If an item is unreasonable as a goal for a patient, he is *dependent* in the skill and should receive Grade 2 dependent. *Example:* Indoor ambulation for a patient with C5-quadriplegia.

211

1. *Not applicable.* The abbreviation N.A. is to be used in the following situations:

   - The item does not apply to this patient because he is too advanced for the activity. *Example:* W/C activities are N.A. for a fully ambulatory patient.
   - Patient does not use the equipment or device asked for in the item.

2. *Dependent.* The patient offers no assistance with the activity. One or more persons may be required for performance of the activity.

3. *Maximal physical assistance.* The patient performs less than one half the work of the activity. Only one person is required for physical assistance.

4. *Moderate physical assistance.* The patient performs approximately one half the work of the activity. Only one person is required for physical assistance.

5. *Minimal physical assistance.* The patient performs more than one half the work of the activity but may require "hands on" or "contact" guarding.

6. *Supervision.* The patient does not require physical assistance or contact to perform the activity. Verbal cueing, demonstration, "hands off" guarding, or "standby" may be necessary. Patient cannot be left alone to perform the activity safely.

7. *Independent.* The patient can be left alone to perform the activity safely and within a reasonable length of time.

AT DISCHARGE ONLY:

Ed. Education to be marked with an (x) for all items the family demonstrates competency in performing, assisting, or supervising.

General Format

This form is a checklist system designed to give a graphic picture of the patient's abilities. The activities are divided into six categories: mobility, balance, W/C independence, transfer independence, ambulatory independence, and equipment. The items in each category are listed in ascending order of difficulty. An (x) should be placed in the box representing the degree of assistance the patient needs to perform the activity.

Spaces have been provided under several of the items that frequently require equipment or where notation of distance is indicated. If no equipment is used, record "none." Record distance in units of feet or yards. Do not leave a blank space.

Example:

	1	2	3	4	5	6	7
W/C ←→ toilet transfer						x	
equipment used				raised seat			

	1	2	3	4	5	6	7
indoor W/C propulsion							x
distance				350 feet			

Lines have been provided at the end of each category for any further explanation or detail. Make any comments pertinent to the performance of the items listed in that category that will give the reader a clearer picture of the patient's function. *Date the comments.*

Interpretations of the Items

Many of the items listed on the form are self explanatory and require no further description. The items on the form that are preceded by an asterisk (*) will be described below. These are the criteria to be examined when determining a patient's functional level. This will help assure the department that all staff members are evaluating the patients based on the same set of criteria.

Mobility

- *bed mobility*—all the items listed under bed mobility are to be tested on a *bed*, not on a raised mat table.
- *rise from supine to short sitting*—patient must rise from the supine position to sitting with both legs over the edge of the bed.
- *move on bed*—patient must be able to move from side to side and up and down in the bed.
- *move on floor*—patient must be able to move in all directions on the floor. (*Example:* Could the patient move away from a dangerous situation such as a hot radiator?)
- *knee walking*—patient must be able to knee walk in all directions (forward, backward, sideways), or it must be noted otherwise on the lines below the category.

W/C Independence

- *weight shift*—this is to test the patient's ability to use some effective method of pressure relief in the

W/C. Note on the lines below the category the method of relief, such as forward lean or lateral shift, if the McCormick loops were used, or if elevating armrests, Medicliner, push-up, and so on were necessary.

- *lock and unlock brakes*—note the use of brake extensions on the lines below if they are necessary for the activity.

- *manage footrests*—patient must be able to place feet on the floor, take off or swing away footrest (whichever is necessary for the individual's function), place the footrests in a position where they can be reached for replacing, and replace footrests in position for use. Raising and lowering legrest should be included if applicable.

- *manage armrests*—patient must be able to unlock, take off and replace armrest, and lock the armrest in position. Include the operation of elevating armrest if applicable.

- *indoor propulsion*—includes propelling forward and backward, turning right and left, turning around a corner to the right and left, maneuvering in small areas, and propelling the W/C on carpeting. The distance listed below refers to *forward distance*. List special equipment such as projections, plastic coated handrims, and electric drive on the lines below the category.

- *manage doors*—patient must be able to open the door, pass through, and close the door. Include doors that open toward and away from the individual and round door knobs.

- *maneuver outdoors*—patient is to be evaluated on grass, concrete, gravel, and rough terrain (broken sidewalk).

- *inclines*—patient is to be evaluated going up and down the 1:10 ratio incline. If a steeper incline is possible, note this on the lines below. Also note if the ramp retarder is used.

- *curb jumping*—patient is to be evaluated going up and down a four-inch curb. If another height curb is possible, note this on the lines below the category, but mark the box for this category based on performance of a four-inch curb.

- cross street safely—include the patient's ability to look to both sides, to judge the distance and time required to cross that distance, and to attend to traffic signals, distances, and oncoming traffic.

- *negotiates elevators*—patient must be able to press the button to call for the elevator, manage the doors, safely propel into the elevator, press the button for destination, and maneuver out of the elevator.

Transfer Independence

- In order to be graded as independent, the patient must be able to approach the transfer surface, lock and unlock the W/C, manage the footrests, armrests, seat belts, and equipment, as well as move from surface to surface without help. Indicate the type of transfer used (standing pivot, lateral, or front) on the lines below the category.

- *W/C←→car*—note on the lines below the category whether the transfer was to the passenger or driver side of the car. Patient must be able to open and close the car door for "independence" in this activity.

- *W/C←→armless chair*—the chair must have a firm seat and no arms.

- *W/C←→upholstered furniture*—an upholstered couch, sofa, or chair may be used for evaluation of this item.

Ambulatory Independence

- *armless chair←→standing*—use a chair with a firm seat and no arms.

- *upholstered furniture←→standing*—an upholstered couch, sofa, or chair may be used for this item.

- *walk forward*—do not include walking on carpeting. If the patient can walk on carpeting, note this on the lines below the category. (Parallel bars may be the equipment used upon initial ambulation assessment only, unless patient never progresses out of the parallel bars.)

- *manage doors*—the patient must be able to open the door, pass through, and close the door. Include doors that open toward and away from the individual.

- *step over obstacles*—use obstacles approximately two inches in height for this test.

- *manages inclines*—the patient must be able to go up and down the 1:5 ratio incline.

- *outdoor ambulation*—distance here refers to *forward distance* only. Patient is to be evaluated on grass, concrete, gravel, and rough terrain (broken sidewalks).

- *stairs with and without railings*—it is usually not necessary to do any more than two flights (average eight steps to a flight). Grade this item based on performance on six-inch stairs only.
- *curbs*—patient must be able to step up and down six-inch curbs. If another size curb is possible, note that on the lines below the category.
- *cross street safely*—patient walks across the street looking in both directions, attending to the traffic signals, judging distances, oncoming traffic, and crosses within a reasonable amount of time.
- *elevator*—the patient must be able to press the button to call for the elevator, manage the doors, walk into the elevator, press the button for destination, and walk out of the elevator safely.
- *escalator*—patient can mount and dismount escalator as well as steady self while riding it.
- *public transportation*—patient can pay the fair, take a seat, walk while the vehicle is in motion, call for appropriate stop, and enter and exit safely.

KEY TO THE RESPIRATORY EVALUATION FORM (EXHIBIT F–3)

Usage

All inpatients should be considered for a respiratory evaluation using all or part of the form, as appropriate.

If respiratory goals have been set during the inpatient admission, the form should be completed again on the recheck evaluation.

Outpatients should be considered for a respiratory evaluation and the form filled out, if respiratory goals are indicated.

Purpose

The form upon completion should reflect the expected competence of the patient's pulmonary status and indicate areas in which goals to upgrade that status can be set.

Source of Data

Objective Tests

Objective tests are to be obtained by the therapist by testing or measuring at the time of the evaluation. Information must not be recorded on the basis of information from the medical record or on the basis of patient/"responsible other" testimony.

Subjective Tests

A and D can be obtained by observation, by testing at the time of the evaluation, or from the medical record or a history from the patient and/or "responsible other."

B and C can be obtained by the therapist by observation, except for GPB, which is to be tested by measuring the vital capacity.

Frequency of Testing

Testing should be performed at time of admission and discharge. Interim testing of parts or the whole of the evaluation should be done as appropriate. Objective tests at discharge must be retested or measured and recorded. Subjective tests where appropriate can be recorded as "no change since initial evaluation."

Position

- sup. = patient is supine on cart or bed or exercise mat when the evaluation is being done.
- sit. = patient is sitting in W/C or on an exercise mat or in bed, with or without support when the evaluation is being done.
- stand. = patient is standing with or without support when the evaluation is being done.

Abdominal Support

Note whether or not the patient is wearing an abdominal binder at the time of the evaluation.

Abbreviations

- *N/A*—used if the patient has bulbar involvement or such muscular incoordination that the test cannot be performed or if the patient cannot cognitively cooperate with the tests. An open tracheostomy may preclude some of the tests in some cases. The reason for not giving the test is to be stated on the form.
- *N/T*—used if time does not allow or if patient refuses the test. State the reason for writing N/T.
- *N/C*—used under subjective tests only where history and observation show no change.

Objective Tests

(must be retested and status indicated even if they show no change)

Vital Capacity

Patient takes in the biggest breath he can, holds the air, then blows it into the spirometer. GPB may be used using three maneuvers for each maximum breath. State that GPB was used, and its use must be consistent at each testing. A reading is taken of three breaths performed as above and the best of the three is documented. Patient may be given assistance in holding the spirometer. No other physical assist is given.

Vital Capacity Expected Normal

Patient's age and body weight are noted and chart referred to for obtaining this reading for a person with intact musculature.

Tidal Volume

Patient breathes into the spirometer in a relaxed normal breathing pattern for 10 breaths in and out. The reading on the spirometer is taken and divided by 10. This gives the tidal volume. On spirometers that do not record below 1,000 liters, start with needle on the 1,000 mark, take away 1,000 and divide by 10 as above.

Respiratory Rate

To be counted when patient is at rest and relaxed and has not done anything within a five-minute time span. This count is preferably done without the patient's knowledge.

Phonation

Count number of syllables patient can produce using normal tidal volume in as normal a situation as can be reproduced (i.e., patient is relaxed and has not exerted himself within a five-minute time span). This count is also preferably done without the patient's knowledge.

Cough

Patient takes in the biggest breath he can and forcefully expels it. If GPB is used, this is recorded with the number of maneuvers.

- *Dependent* refers to a patient who has paralysis of all respiratory muscles or who is unable to coordinate their muscle power to take air in and/or expel it with any functional force, even with the assistance of another person.
- *Assist* indicates that patient and/or responsible other needs to give pressure to substitute for lack of abdominal musculature in order to produce an effective cough.
- *Independent* indicates that patient can produce an effective cough and move secretions as necessary at will, including those patients who use self-assistive techniques.

Chest Expansion

Patient takes in the biggest breath he can and measurement of this is taken. The rib cage is measured at the xiphoid process. If GPB is used to get the biggest breath, note this with the number of maneuvers used.

Subjective Tests

Chest Formation

With patient *unclothed,* note and record what you see in bony structure, tendon and muscle structure. Palpate for muscle tone with or without movement as indicated and make a note of which way it was done.

Breathing Pattern

With patient *unclothed* and at rest, note chest movement and muscles used to produce movement and record. If patient was exerted and then breathing pattern noted, record that patient was exerted. Note if patient uses GPB in either of the above situations. Note breath sounds if abnormal. Note if patient uses accessory muscles and, if so, when and which muscles.

Cough Effectiveness

Ask patient to take the biggest breath in that he can and forcefully expel it. Record how forceful it sounded, how loud or soft, deep or shallow, if it took a long time to expel the breath. If GPB was used and if so, how many maneuvers to produce the breath. Was the cough productive? If it was, describe secretions, viscous or fluid, smell, if any, color, and amount.

Other Observations

Get all relevant respiratory history from patient, significant other, or patient's medical chart. Observe and record if significant: color of lips, color and shape of nails, if patient smokes (note how many, how often), if patient is brain damaged if this is significant to the respiratory evaluation, and if patient has any bulbar involvement.

Exhibit F–1 Muscle Examination Form

MUSCLE EXAMINATION

Patient's Name _____ RIC Number _____

Date of Birth _____ Date of Onset _____

Diagnosis _____

Left   Right

					Examiner's Initials						
					Date						
			NECK	Flexors	Sternocleidomastoid (st.)	Accessory	C 1-3				
					Sternocleidomastoid (cl.)	Accessory	C 1-3				
					Extensor group		C 1-6				
			TRUNK	Flexors	Upper rectus abdominis		T 7-10				
					Lower rectus abdominis		T10-L1				
				R Ext. obl.	Rotators { L Ext. obl.		T 7-10				
				L Int. obl.	{ R Int. obl.		T 7-10				
				Extensors	Thoracic group		T 1-9				
					Lumbar group		T10-L5				
				Pelvic elev.	Quadratus Lumborum		T12-L2				
			HIP	Flexors	Iliopsoas	Femoral	L 1-4				
				Extensors	Gluteus maximus	Inf. Glut.	L 5-S2				
				Abductors	Gluteus Medius	Sup. Glut.	L 4-S1				
				Adductor group		Obturator	L 2-S1				
				External rotator group			L 3-S2				
				Internal rotator group			L 4-S2				
				Sartorius		Femoral	L 2-4				
				Tensor fasciae latae		Sup. Glut.	L 4-S1				
			KNEE	Flexors	Biceps femoris	Sciatic	L 5-S3				
					Inner hamstrings	Sciatic	L 5-S2				
				Extensors	Quadriceps	Femoral	L 2-L4				
			ANKLE	Plantar flexors	Gastrocnemius	Tibial	S 1-2				
					Soleus	Tibial	S 1-2				
			FOOT	Invertors	Tibialis anterior	D. Peroneal	L 4-S1				
					Tibialis posterior	Tibial	L 5-S2				
				Evertors	Peroneus brevis	Sup. Peroneal	L 4-S1				
					Peroneus longus	Sup. Peroneal	L 4-S1				
			TOES	M.P. Flexors	Lumbricals	Tibial	L 4-S3				
				P.I.P. Flexors	Flex. digit. brevis	Med. Plantar	L 4-S1				
				D.I.P. Flexors	Flex. digit. longus	Tibial	L 5-S2				
				M.P. Extensors	Ext. digit. longus	D. Peroneal	L 4-S1				
					Ext. digit. brevis	D. Peroneal	L 4-S1				
			HALLUX	M.P. Flexor	Flex. hall. brevis	Plantar	L 4-S2				
				I.P. Flexor	Flex. hall. longus	Tibial	L 5-S2				
				M.P. Extensor	Ext. hall. brevis	D. Peroneal	L 4-S1				
				I.P. Extensor	Ext. hall. longus	D. Peroneal	L 4-S1				

Remarks:

KEY

5	N	Normal	Complete range of motion against gravity with full resistance.	S or SS	Spasm or Severe Spasm
4	G	Good*	Complete range of motion against gravity with some resistance.	C or CC	Contracture or Severe contracture
3	F	Fair*	Complete range of motion against gravity.		
2	P	Poor*	Complete range of motion with gravity eliminated.		
1	T	Trace	Evidence of slight contractility. No joint motion.		
0	0	Zero	No evidence of contractility.		

*Muscle spasm or contracture may limit range of motion. A question mark should be placed after the grading of a movement that is incomplete from this cause.

Exhibit F–1 continued

Left			Group	Action	Muscle	Nerve	Root	Right		
					Date & Examiner's Initials					
			SCAPULA	Abductor	Serratus anterior	Long thoracic	C 5-7			
				Elevator	Upper trapezius	Spinal Accessory	C 3-4			
				Depressor	Lower trapezius	Spinal Accessory	C 3-4			
				Adductors	Middle trapezius	Spinal Accessory	C 3-4			
					Rhomboids	Dorsal scapular	C 4-5			
			SHOULDER	Flexor	Anterior deltoid	Axillary	C 5-6			
				Extensors	Latissimus dorsi	Thoracodorsal	C 6-8			
					Teres major	L. Subscap.	C 5-6			
				Abductor	Middle deltoid	Axillary	C 5-6			
				Horiz. abd.	Posterior deltoid	Axillary	C 5-6			
				Horiz. add.	Pectoralis major	Ant. Thoracic	C 5-T1			
				External rotator group			C 4-T1			
				Internal rotator group			C 4-T1			
			ELBOW	Flexors	Biceps brachii	Musculo.	C 5-6			
					Brachioradialis	Radial	C 5-6			
				Extensor	Triceps	Radial	C 6-8			
			FOREARM	Supinator		Radial	C 6			
				Pronator group - Pron. quad & teres		Radial & Median	C 5-T1			
			WRIST	Flexors	Flex. carpi. rad.	Median	C 6-7			
					Flex. carpi. uln.	Ulnar	C 7-T1			
				Extensors	Ext. carpi. rad. 1. & br.	Radial	C 6-7			
					Ext. carpi. uln.	Radial	C 6-8			
			FINGERS	M.P. Flexors	Lumbricales	1 Median	C 7-T1			
					Lumbricales	2 Median	C 7-T1			
					Lumbricales	3 Ulnar	C 7-T1			
					Lumbricales	4 Ulnar	C 7-T1			
				P.I.P. Flexors-Flex. digit. sub.		1 Median	C 7-T1			
				"		2 Median	C 7-T1			
				"		3 Median	C 7-T1			
				"		4 Median	C 7-T1			
				D.I.P. Flexors-Flex. digit. prof.		1 Median	C 7-T1			
				"		2 Median	C 7-T1			
				"		3 Ulnar	C 7-T1			
				"		4 Ulnar	C 7-T1			
				M.P. Extensor-Ext. digit. comm.		1 Radial	C 6-8			
				"		2 Radial	C 6-8			
				"		3 Radial	C 6-8			
				"		4 Radial	C 6-8			
				Adductors - Palmer Interoseous		1 Ulnar	C 8-T1			
				"		2 Ulnar	C 8-T1			
				"		3 Ulnar	C 8-T1			
				Abductors - Dorsal Interoseous		1 Ulnar	C 8-T1			
				"		2 Ulnar	C 8-T1			
				"		3 Ulnar	C 8-T1			
				"		4 Ulnar	C 8-T1			
				Abductor digiti quinti		Ulnar	C 8-T1			
				Opponens digiti quinti		Ulnar	C 8-T1			
			THUMB	M.P. Flexor	Flex. poll. brevis	Med. & Ulnar	C 6-T1			
				I.P. Flexor	Flex. poll. longus	Med. & Ulnar	C 6-T1			
				M.P. Extensor	Ext. poll. brevis	Radial	C 6-8			
				I.P. Extensor	Ext. poll. longus	Radial	C 6-8			
				Abductors	Abd. poll. brevis	Median	C 8-T1			
					Abd. poll. longus	Radial	C 6-7			
					Adductor pollicis	Ulnar	C 8-T1			
					Opponens pollicis	Median	C 8-T1			

Exhibit F–2 ADL Assessment Form

REHABILITATION INSTITUTE OF CHICAGO
PHYSICAL THERAPY DEPARTMENT
ACTIVITIES OF DAILY LIVING

NAME_____ RIC # _____ BIRTHDATE _____

DIAGNOSIS _____ONSET_____

METHOD OF GRADING

1. Not tested (N/T) or not applicable (N/A)
2. Dependent
3. Maximal physical assistance
4. Moderate physical assistance
5. Minimal physical assistance
6. Supervision
7. Independent
(*) See key for specific description of the item

Mark the appropriate box with an [x] Date

Initials

MOBILITY	1	2	3	4	5	6	7	1	2	3	4	5	6	7	1	2	3	4	5	6	7	Ed
* Bed: roll supine to right sidelying																						
roll supine to left sidelying																						
roll supine to prone																						
roll prone to supine																						
rise from supine to long sitting																						
*rise from supine to short sitting																						
*move on the bed																						
Assume prone on elbows(from prone)																						
Assume supine on elbows(from supine)																						
* Move on the floor																						
Assume elbows and knees																						
Belly crawling																						
Assume hands and knees																						
Creeping on hands and knees																						
Assume kneeling																						
* Knee walking																						

WHEELCHAIR INDEPENDENCE	1	2	3	4	5	6	7	1	2	3	4	5	6	7	1	2	3	4	5	6	7	Ed
*Weight shift in the wheelchair																						
*Lock and unlock brakes																						
*Manage footrests																						
*Manage armrests																						
*Indoor propulsion																						
distance without rest period																						
*Manage doors																						
*Maneuver outdoors																						
distance without rest period																						
*Inclines (1:10)																						
*Curb jumping (4" curbs)																						
*Cross street safely																						
*Manage elevators																						

REV. 3/27/79

Exhibit F–2 continued

*TRANSFER INDEPENDENCE	1	2	3	4	5	6	7	1	2	3	4	5	6	7	1	2	3	4	5	6	7	Ed
W/C ←→ bed																						
equipment used																						
W/C ←→ toilet(transfer only)																						
equipment used																						
W/C ←→ bath(transfer only)																						
equipment used																						
* W/C ←→ car(excluding w/c)																						
W/C ←→ car(including w/c)																						
* W/C ←→ armless chair																						
* W/C ←→ upholstered furniture																						
W/C ←→ floor																						

AMBULATORY INDEPENDENCE	1	2	3	4	5	6	7	1	2	3	4	5	6	7	1	2	3	4	5	6	7	Ed
W/C ←→ standing																						
* Armless chair ←→ standing																						
Bed ←→ standing																						
* Upholstered furniture ←→ standing																						
Toilet ←→ standing																						
equipment used																						
Car ←→ standing																						
Bath ←→ standing																						
equipment used																						
* Walk forward indoors																						
equipment used																						
distance w/o rest period																						
Walk backward (5 feet)																						
Walk sideways (5 feet)																						
* Manage doors																						
* Step over obstacles																						
Pick up object from floor																						
* Manage inclines (1:5)																						
* Stairs with railing																						
# of stairs w/o rest period																						
* Stairs w/o railing																						
# of stairs w/o rest period																						
equipment used																						
* Outdoor ambulation																						
equipment used																						
distance w/o rest period																						
* Curbs (6")																						
* Cross street safely																						
Floor ←→ standing																						
Manage bus step																						
* Manage elevator																						
* Manage escalator																						
* Manage public transportation																						

EQUIPMENT MANAGEMENT	1	2	3	4	5	6	7	1	2	3	4	5	6	7	1	2	3	4	5	6	7	Ed
LE orthosis don and doff																						
Binder or corset don & doff																						
Other:																						

Exhibit F–3 Respiratory Evaluation Form

REHABILITATION INSTITUTE OF CHICAGO
PHYSICAL THERAPY
RESPIRATORY EVALUATION

Patient Name:

RIC Number:

Physician:

Date:

DIAGNOSIS/IMPAIRMENT _____

DATE OF ONSET OF IMPAIRMENT: _____

DATE OF BIRTH _____

☐ Inpatient   ☐ Outpatient

(All therapists see KEY for description of items:)

N/A - Not applicable
N/T - Not tested
NC - No change

Examiners Name				
Date				
Position (Sup., Sit, Stand)				
Abdominal Support?				

I. OBJECTIVE TESTS

A. Vital Capacity (Liters)				
B. Vital Capacity (expected normal) (Fill in expected normal V.C. for individual with intact musculature)				
C. Tidal Volume (Liters)				
D. Respiratory Rate (Breaths/Minute)				
E. Phonation (Syllables/Breath)				
F. Cough (dependent, assist, independent)				
B. Chest Expansion (Centimeters) (measured at ziphoid process)				

II. SUBJECTIVE TESTS

	Date	Date
	Initial Evaluation	Discharge Evaluation
A. Chest Formation: (Shape, symmetry, bony abnormalities, muscle tone, atrophy)		
B. Breathing Pattern: (diaphragmatic, accessory muscles, segmental breathing, breath sounds, tracheostomy glossopharyngeal breathing		
C. Cough Effectiveness: (Force, timing, sound, productivity)		
D. Other observations: (Significant respiratory history, smoking, color, brain damage considerations,etc.)		

RIC 1-01255 10 (3/81)

Exhibit F–4 Home Assessment Form

The Home Assessment Evaluation is a tool for physical and occupational therapists to plan the ADL program, order appropriate equipment and make suggestions for changes necessary for the patient to function in the home.

The patient will be given this form to fill out by the time of the second home pass. Family members should help to measure and should participate.

All appropriate questions should be answered and the form returned to the physical therapist so that plans for discharge can be made.

NAME _____

HOSPITAL NO. _____

HOME ADDRESS _____

PHYSICAL THERAPIST _____

OCCUPATIONAL THERAPIST _____

DATE _____

HOME ASSESSMENT FORM

I. General Information
   A. Type of financial coverage
   B. Type of home:
      One-story ___ Two-story ___
      Apt. ___ Floor ___
      No. of stairs between floors ___
      Railings: L ___ R ___
      Front door width ___
      Threshold height ___
      No. of stairs to front door ___
         height ___
      No. of stairs to back door ___
         height ___
      Back door width ___
      Threshold height ___
      Elevator available ___
      Own ___ Rent ___ Other ___
      Can remodeling be done? ___
   C. No. of people living in home ___
      Are there pets? ___ Children? ___

RECOMMENDATIONS:

II. Outside
   A. Driveway: Location _____
      Surface type: ___ Inclined ___
   B. Parking: Location _____
      Can patient transfer in and out of car? ___
   C. Walkway: Location _____
      Surface type _____
   D. Entry: Can patient enter alone? ___
      One assist ___ Two assist ___
      In emergency can patient get out alone? ___
      Is adequate assistance available? ___
III. Bedroom:
   A. Can patient maneuver into bedroom? ___
      Door width ___ Threshold height ___
   B. Bed: Type of bed _____
      Height: Top of mattress to floor ___
      Can patient transfer into bed? ___
      If no, why? _____
         Approaches bed: R ___ L ___

For transfers and dressing:
Mattress is adequately firm ___
Railings needed ___
Mattress width ___
Would hospital bed fit in room?
   ___ Standard (36″ × 80″)
   ___ Extra long (36″ × 84″)
   C. Clothing: Accessible to patient
      Closet ___ Drawers ___
   D. Accessible light switch at bedside and doorway ___
   Please draw a diagram of bedroom on the back of this page showing layout and dimensions.

RECOMMENDATIONS:

IV. Bathroom:
   A. Door entrance width ___
      Threshold height ___
      Accessible light switch ___
   Is adequate maneuvering space available?
   Alone ___ Assisted ___
   B. Tub approach:
      R ___ L ___ Head-on ___
      Can patient transfer in and out of the tub? ___
      Equipment used for transferring in and out of tub: _____
      Tub design:
      Standard ___ Round bottomed w/legs ___
      Height ___ Inside flat width ___
      Glass door ___ Can it be removed? ___
      Type of wall _____
      Faucets accessible _____
      Shower head height _____
   C. Shower stall:
      Height of ledge ___
      Stall dimensions ___
      Is floor level? ___
      Height of shower head ___
      Type of wall ___
      Turn faucets on ___ off ___
   D. Sink:
      Turn faucets on ___ off ___
      Describe type _____

Exhibit F–4 continued

Knee space under sink ___
Exposed pipes padded under sink ___
Mirror adequate level for patient ___
Accessible storage area ___
Accessible electric outlet ___
Accessible towel rack ___
E. Toilet:
Seat height ___
Can patient transfer on and off toilet? ___
Tank present ___ Stable ___
Distance between holes for toilet seat bolts: ___
Inches of available space: R ___ L ___
Please draw a diagram of bathroom on the back of this form, showing layout and dimensions.

RECOMMENDATIONS:

V. Kitchen:
A. General: Door width ___
Floor covering ___
Pantry and shelves accessible ___
Accessible light switch ___
Accessible electrical outlets ___
Adequate maneuvering space available: ___
B. Stove:
Height from floor to burner surface ___
Oven location ___
Can patient put in and remove food? ___
Location of controls ___
Gas ___ Electric ___ Automatic pilot ___
Is counter space available? ___
Can observation mirror be installed? ___
C. Sink:
Height from floor ___
Number of basins ___
Stainless steel ___ Porcelain ___
Type of faucets ___
Turn faucets on ___ off ___
Will W/C fit under sink? ___
Any exposed pipes? ___
Spray nozzle available ___
Garbage disposal ___
Type of on/off switch ___
Location of switch ___
Counter space available: R ___ L ___
D. Can patient carry food or hot item to table? ___
E. Cabinets:
Open easily ___
Overhead ___ Under counter ___
Accessibility: Food ___ Dishes ___ Utensils ___
Reorganization necessary ___
F. Refrigerator: ___
Location ___
Hinges on L ___ R ___
Opens and closes easily ___
Freezer location ___
Food accessible ___
Counter accessible ___
G. Kitchen table:
W/C fits under ___
Workspace available ___

H. Dishwasher:
Top load ___ Front load ___
Arrangements for grocery shopping: ___
Please draw diagram of kitchen on the back of this form, showing layout and dimensions.

RECOMMENDATIONS:

VI. Laundry:
Location ___
Stairs ___ Rails ___
Door width ___ Threshold ___
Accessible light switch ___
Accessible electrical outlets ___
Accessible: Washer ___ Dryer ___ Wringer ___
Ironing board ___

RECOMMENDATIONS:

VII. Miscellaneous
A. Telephone location ___
Accessible from: Floor ___
W/C ___
B. Hallways: Can W/C be maneuvered into and between rooms? ___
C. Flooring type ___
D. Are there any throw rugs? ___
E. Can patient maneuver around furniture easily? ___
F. Can patient open windows? ___
G. Are heat controls available? ___
H. Can patient work controls of TV? ___
Radio ___ Other ___
I. Can patient open all doors? ___
J. Is there a way for contacting help in an emergency? ___
K. Is help available? Day ___ Night ___
VIII. Employment:
A. Present goals and plans:

B. Job description:

C. Transportation to work ___
D. Accessibility of:
Washroom ___ Cafeteria ___
Telephone or emergency help ___
E. Equipment needed:

IX. School:
A. Name and address of school:

B. Will patient be living at school? ___
C. Accessibility of: Washrooms ___
Cafeteria ___ Telephone ___
Library ___ Classrooms ___
D. Can patient manage the following? Locker ___
Books ___ Notetaking ___ Elevators ___

RECOMMENDATIONS:

Exhibit F–5 Exercise Class Form

NAME OF CLASS: _____

NAME OF PATIENT: _____ HOSPITAL NO. _____

PHYSICIAN'S NAME _____ STARTING DATE _____

DIAGNOSIS: _____ DAYS SCHEDULED _____

PRECAUTIONS _____

—FILL IN WITH APPROPRIATE DATE ANY CHANGE IN STATUS—

INDEPENDENCE _____

MOTIVATION _____

JUDGMENT _____

COMMUNICATION SKILLS _____

PERCEPTUAL PROBLEMS _____

ASSISTIVE DEVICES (1) CANE (list type) _____

(2) ORTHOSIS (list type and setting) _____

_____

GOALS: _____

_____

THERAPIST: _____

Exhibit F–6 Therapeutic Pool Record

NAME:			HOSPITAL NO.
INPATIENT OUTPATIENT	AGE	PHYSICIAN	
DIAGNOSIS:			
DISABILITY:			
PRECAUTIONS:			
GOALS:			
TREATMENT:			
COMMENTS:			

Bibliography and Reading List

Accessibility

Accessibility Standards—State of Illinois, 1978. Available free from Capital Development Board, State of Illinois, 180 N. LaSalle Street #320, Chicago, IL 60601.

An Accessible Entrance: Ramps, 1979. Available from Design Coalition, Inc., 1201 Williamson Street, Madison, WI 53703.

An Accessible Bathroom, 1980. Available from Design Coalition, Inc.,1201 Williamson Street, Madison, WI 53703.

Catlin, J. *Adaptable Housing.* Booklet available from Access Living of Metropolitan Chicago, 505 N. LaSalle, Chicago, IL 60610.

Cary, J. R. 1978. *How to create interiors for the disabled: A guidebook for family and friends.* New York: Pantheon Books.

Autonomic Dysreflexia

Erickson, R. P. 1980. Autonomic hyperreflexia: Pathology and medical management. *Arch. Phys. Med. Rehab.* 61:431–440.

Taylor, A. G. 1974. Autonomic dysreflexia in spinal cord injury. *Nursing Clin. North Am.* 9:4.

Linden, R. et al. 1980. Incidence and clinical features of autonomic dysreflexia in patients with spinal cord injuries. *Paraplegia* 18:285–292.

Ectopic Bone

Chantrine, A., and Minaire, P. 1981. Para-osteo-arthropathies. *J. Rehab. Med. Scand.* 13:1, 31–37.

FES

Baker, L. L. et al. 1980. *Functional electrical stimulation: A practical clinical guide.* Downey, Ca.: Association of Ranchos Los Amigos.

Gait

Abramson, A. S. 1948. Bone disturbances in injuries to the spinal cord and cauda equina (paraplegia). *J. Bone Joint Surg. [Am]* 30:982–987.

Abramson, A. S., and Delagi, E. F. 1960. Influence of weight-bearing and muscle contraction on disuse osteoporosis. *Arch. Phys. Med. Rehabil.* 42:147–151.

Bergmann, et al. 1977–1978. Study of calcium and bone metabolism in paraplegic patients. *Paraplegia* 15147–15159.

Cerny, K., Waters, R., Hislop, H., and Perry, J. 1980. Walking and wheelchair energetics in persons with paraplegia. *Phys. Ther.* 60:1133–1139.

Claus-Walker, J., Campos, R. J., Carter, E. R. et al. 1972. Calcium excretion in quadriplegia. *Arch. Phys. Med. Rehabil.* 53:14–20.

Huitt, C. T., and Gwyer, J. L. 1978. Paraplegic ambulatory training using Craig-Scott orthoses. *Phys. Ther.* 58:8:976–978.

Hussey, R. W., and Stauffer, E. S. 1973. Spinal cord injury: Requirements for ambulation. *Arch. Phys. Med. Rehabil.* 54:544.

Kaplan, P. E., Gandhavadi, B., Richards, L., and Goldschmidt, J. 1978. Calcium balance in paraplegic patients: Influence of injury duration and ambulation. *Arch. Phys. Med. Rehabil.* 59:447–450.

Mikelberg, R., and Reid, S. 1981. Spinal cord lesions and lower extremity bracing: An overview and follow-up study. *Paraplegia* 19:379–385.

Quigley, M. J. 1977. Should functional ambulation be a goal for paraplegic persons? *Orthotics Pros. Newsletter* 4–6.

Medical

Burke, D. C., and Murray, D. D. 1975. *Handbook of spinal cord medicine.* New York: Macmillan.

Calenoff, L., ed. 1981. *Radiology of spinal cord injury.* St. Louis: Mosby.

Guttman, L. 1976. *Spinal cord injuries: Comprehensive management and research.* 2nd ed. London: Blackwell Scientific Publications.

Hoppenfeld, S. 1976. *Physical examination of the spine and extremities.* New York: Appleton-Century-Crofts.

Pierce, D. S., and Nickel, V. H. 1977. *Total care of spinal cord injuries.* Boston: Little Brown.

Windie, W. F., ed. 1980. *Spinal cord and its reaction to traumatic injury.* New York: Marcel Dekker.

Posture

Zarkowski, D. 1984. *Wheelchair posture and pressure sores.* Springfield, Ill.: Charles C Thomas.

Pressure Relief

Cochran, G. V. B. 1980. Development of test methods for evaluation of wheelchair cushions. *Bull. Pros. Res.* 17:1, 9–30.

Noble, P. C. The prevention of pressure sores in persons with spinal cord injuries. New York: International Exchange of Information in Rehabilitation, 1981 (monograph)

Psychosocial

Trieschmann, R. B. 1980. *Spinal cord injuries: Psychological, social, and vocational adjustment.* New York: Pergamon Press.

Respiratory

Alvarez, S. E., Peterson, M., and Lunsford, B. R. 1981. Respiratory treatment of the adult patient with spinal cord injury. *Phys. Ther.* 61:112, 1737–1745.

Frownfelter, D. L., ed. 1978. *Chest physical therapy and pulmonary rehabilitation.* Chicago: Year Book Medical Publishers.

Haas, A., Lowman, E. W., and Bergofsky, E. H. 1965. Impairment of respiration after spinal cord injury. *Arch. Phys. Med. Rehabil.* 46:399–405.

Ledsome, J. R., and Sharp, J. M. 1981. Pulmonary function in acute cervical cord injury. *Am. Rev. Respir. Dis.* 124:41–44.

McKinley, A. C., Auchincloss, J. H., Jr., Gilbert, R., and Nicholas, J. J. October 1969. Pulmonary function, ventilatory control, and respiratory complications in quadriplegic subjects. *Am. Rev. Respir. Dis.* 526–532.

Morris, J. F., Koski, A., and Johnson, L. C. 1971. Spirometric standards for healthy non-smoking adults. *Am. Rev. Resp. Dis.* 103:57.

Silver, J. R., and Moulton, A. 1969. The physiological and pathological sequelae of paralysis of intercostal and abdominal muscles in tetraplegic patients. *Paraplegia* 7:131–141. (Paper read at the 1968 scientific meeting)

Sexuality

Mooney, T. et al. 1975. *Sexual options for paraplegics and quadriplegics.* Boston: Little Brown.

Rabin, B. 1980. *The sensuous wheeler.* San Francisco: Multimedia Resource Center.

Shaked, A, ed. 1981. *Human sexuality and rehabilitation medicine (sexual functioning following spinal cord injury).* Baltimore: Williams & Wilkins.

Slings

Johnson, M. M., and Charles, D. B. 1971. Sling suspension techniques, demonstrating the use of a portable frame, Part I. *Phys. Ther.* 51:524–534.

Johnson, M. M., and Charles, D. B. 1971. Sling suspension techniques, demonstrating the use of a portable frame, Part II. *Phys. Ther.* 51:1092–1099.

Johnson, M. M., and Charles, D. B. 1971. Sling suspension techniques, demonstrating the use of a portable frame, Part III. *Phys. Ther.* 51:1288–1998.

Johnson, M. M., and Charles, D. B. 1973. Sling suspension techniques, demonstrating the use of a portable frame, Part IV. *Phys. Ther.* 53:856–862.

Treatment Options and Approaches

Bedbrook, G. 1981. *The care and management of spinal cord injuries.* New York: Springer-Verlag.

Bromley, I. 1981. *Tetraplegia and paraplegia: A guide for physiotherapists,* 2nd ed. New York: Churchill-Livingstone.

Ford, J. R., and Duckworth, B. 1974. *Physical management for the quadriplegic patient.* Philadelphia: Davis.

Sullivan, P. E., Markos, P. D., and Minor, M. A. D. 1982. *An integrated approach to therapeutic exercise: Theory and clinical application.* Reston, Va.: Reston Publishing Co.

Veer, C. *Physiotherapy for tetraplegics and paraplegics,* 1978. Available from Paraplegic Association (CANTY), Inc., P.O. Box 1671, Christchurch, New Zealand (NZ $19.80).

Index

Note: Page numbers in *italics* indicate tables and illustrations.

THE REHABILITATION INSTITUTE OF CHICAGO PUBLICATION SERIES

Don A. Olson, Ph.D., Series Coordinator

Spinal Cord Injury: A Guide to Functional Outcomes in Physical Therapy Management

Stroke/Head Trauma: A Guide to Functional Outcomes in Physical Therapy Management

Lower Extremity Amputation: A Guide to Functional Outcomes in Physical Therapy Management

Clinical Management of Right Hemisphere Dysfunction

Evaluation Protocol for Dysphagia